THIRTY MORE CHIC DAYS

Creating an inspired mindset for a magical life

FIONA FERRIS

ISBN: 9781723722899

Dedication

This book is for my dad, who passed away just before it was published, at the age of 73. He died of a heart attack between races at the Bonneville Salt Flats, USA. Photos taken only a few hours before showed a man doing what he loved – challenging himself to better his previous year's motorcycle speed record.

Pa, you are an inspiration to be someone who lives their life to the fullest. You never considered age a hindrance to fulfilling your dreams. Love you.

Other books by Fiona Ferris

Thirty Chic Days: *Practical inspiration for a beautiful life*

Thirty Slim Days: *Create your slender and healthy life in a fun and enjoyable way*

Financially Chic: *Live a luxurious life on a budget, learn to love managing money, and grow your wealth*

How to be Chic in the Winter: *Living slim, happy and stylish during the cold season*

A Chic and Simple Christmas: *Celebrate the holiday season with ease and grace*

Contents

Day 1
Embrace your inner French girl and her dream life

The idealistic thought of my Paris dream girl encourages me to avoid settling for mediocrity in my closet. She inspires me to drink my coffee black because it is Paris café chic and not because I am trying to cut back on dairy for my sinuses. Seriously, which image would motivate you more?

My inner French girl inspires me like no other, even though I admit I have been slightly embarrassed by her. I felt that real French people might look down their nose at me and sneer, 'She doesn't know what it means to be French' in their divinely sensual accent. And self-conscious that people will think I am pathetic for being inspired by the light skimming of a culture I did not grow up in.

But the heart wants what the heart wants. And my heart implores me to indulge in my faux-French dreams. She wants me to play French music from across the decades including Zaz, Édith Piaf, Carla Bruni, Charles Trenet, Josephine Baker and Madeleine Peyroux. She wants me to watch Woody Allen's *Midnight in Paris* movie and swoon over the colours of the city – beige stone buildings and cobbled streets, red awnings and Paris Métro signs, black art nouveau wrought iron and green park benches.

My heart swells when I think of my alter ego living her chic life in a bijou Parisian apartment; playing an album on her turntable; popping out in jeans and a sharply cut blazer to meet her beau for a glass of champagne at a stylish bistro. Of course her jeans size is tiny and she wears heels even if it is a hot afternoon (because my Paris girl's feet and ankles *never* swell up like mine do).

This has been my life's work (and please don't think me too shallow) – reconciling my Paris daydreams with my real life; shelving all those practical naysayers who say that I shouldn't have my French fantasy life because I don't speak the language and have no desire to live there.

Who's to say what is right anyway? I think the sign of a mature emotional capacity is to carry on with what you love and know is your true path. And Paris? She is one of mine.

I visit Paris via Google Maps sometimes. I'll choose a neighbourhood and take a walk with Street View. If

I'm reading a book that mentions 'Place Pigalle', I'll go and have a look.

I'll watch a French subtitled movie and immerse myself in the feeling of living there. It doesn't matter that I love my life here in New Zealand and will likely never move to France; I can still enjoy and be inspired by my best girl Paris.

Fill yourself up

These sorts of things feed my soul, and when I'm feeding my soul I'm not looking for nourishment or fun elsewhere – namely the snack food aisle of my supermarket. When I am feeding my soul with what thrills me, I feel full, replete and sated.

I play my music around the house, dress in a way that feels chic to me and take the time to shape my eyebrows. I elevate self-care to a whole new level, from lazy and unmotivated to... Paris girl.

Paris girl cannot be tempted with junky chocolate in giant-sized bars when she could savour something altogether more bewitching such as the darkest 90% cacao chocolate which almost tastes like fudge it's so rich. One square at a time is all her senses can handle yet she happily partakes daily.

She loves life and indulges in pleasures every day, but this does not mean eating to excess. She knows her stomach doesn't agree when she does this, and she especially does not like the feeling of her clothes being too tight.

When the waistband starts feeling constrictive, she looks at what she's been eating the past few weeks and adjusts accordingly. Paris girl delights in creating simple, delicious and healthy meals for herself and her beau.

She loves to celebrate too, whether it's a special drink on a Friday or a deliciously early bedtime between pristine sheets on a weeknight. Contrary to what people might think, Paris girl is not out partying all the time. *Non*, she takes good care of herself. She wants to look and feel her best and knows that under-eye circles do not become her.

Paris girl edits her wardrobe and all her possessions on a seasonal basis. At the beginning of the two main seasons she looks at clothes she has saved from last year. She considers whether she still loves them. Some items are put on probation and some remain absolute favourites.

She loves to feel happy in her outfits and is ruthless when it comes to curating her wardrobe. If an item bothers her, she considers why that is. Perhaps the fabric doesn't feel nice or she has erred on the side of *frumpfort* (yes, that's when comfortable meets frumpy). She is usually brilliantly discerning when choosing clothes, but sometimes mistakes will slip through.

Paris girl does value comfort, but not *too much*. She prefers the comfort of her jeans fitting versus the comfort of a pair of elastic-waist track pants. Elastic-waist track pants worn daily are at the top of a slippery slope to Nibblesville and she has no desire to visit there.

She is not too precious either. She loves to add kitsch touches into her life, whether it's a celebrity perfume, leopard-print knickers or pulling her hair into a high ponytail.

Paris girl enjoys being inspired by other cultures and has a special place in her heart for the US of A with its can-do attitude and timeless sportswear heritage.

She staves off staidness and keeps herself youthful by picking up small personal style details that appeal to her on others. She keeps her ears open for new music and the latest app. She doesn't take on everything for herself but delights in keeping in touch and knowing what is happening around her.

Her greatest fear is staying the same, never changing. She doesn't want to let herself become stiff or stale. She wants to be unpredictable, interesting and free.

Invite her in

It doesn't matter that she doesn't exist in real life because she can exist in *your* life, starting with your mind. And who wouldn't be inspired by a creature as entrancing as her? Does she need to walk down the street and allow you to touch her slender arm to know that she is real?

My Paris girl motivates me in an effortless way. She powers me towards my dream way of living simply by being. She is fleeting and ethereal in my mind, and that's why I am so entranced by her. As she steps down the Avenue des Champs-Élysées and around a corner to duck into her favourite boutique, I lose sight of her again. She's always one step ahead of me, showing me the way.

That girl, she is something else. She is my love though, my life. Because she is me. I am that girl. I have that lifestyle and those dreams. Deep inside I am her. She leads me, feeds me and completes me.

Surely now you must understand that to ignore her in favour of being reasonable and practical is to ignore your own pleasure and happiness. When you try to 'grow up' and put her in her proper place it's as if a light has been switched off. She illuminates you from the inside out.

I am so grateful for her. That, my friends, is why I cannot ever give her up. I must protect her with my daydreams and fanciful thoughts because she is my *raison d'etre* – my reason for living.

If we don't have our inner life, we have nothing. Everything comes from within and we must nurture that secret garden that dwells inside each of us.

Who is your girl? What does she love? What lifts her heart and makes her smile? Could you do more for her?

Please don't ignore that voice; she needs you to listen. When you don't tune your ear for her you will look for pleasure in other ways and this will be a faux pleasure. Trust me, I know. My faux pleasure was industrial quantities of chocolate and other sweet foods.

Trucking this into my mouth *en masse* did not fill me up. That hunger was endless and could not be allayed with food. It was only when I reacquainted myself with my inner me, the chic Paris me, that I felt whole again.

When I dared look in her direction she said nothing, but simply took me by the hand and squeezed it tight. *Bonjour my friend, I've missed you*, she whispered as we strolled off.

Thirty Chic Days inspirational ideas:

Who is this girl for you? Was she there for you as a teen or younger, or as an adult? What does she love and what would she die for? How would she feed you, both body and mind, and what clothes would she have you wear?

Write down all your many and varied influences, daydreams and favourite words, reaching back as far as you need to. When you feel a thrill inside, that's when you'll know you are onto something. Chase that feeling and note down all the ideas that make you feel happy.

What would she say if you invited her over to your home for a visit? Picture her coming through the front door and looking around. Put yourself in her shoes, her eyes, and view your home that way. See if there are ways where you are not fully allowing yourself to be all of her... all of you.

Indulge in her fantasy life and see how everything becomes brighter, more golden, happier and fun. Live life with her and please remember to bring her along. She needs you and you need her. She is your lifelong best friend and confidant. She will always be there for you.

Day 2
Choose glamour

I consider myself a practical person who has chosen the hardest-wearing, easiest-care option for most things I've ever purchased. I've worked out that mid-tones are the perfect choice for expensive long-term items such carpet, drapes and sofas etc. Why? Because too light and they'll show the dirt easily, too dark and they will fade or show fluff. Our home (and my closet) is a symphony of mid-tones.

And yet, there is a side of me that is lured to the glamour. To an all-white home punctuated with sparkling crystal and mirrored surfaces. Or the mystery of a room painted in a deep, dark shade.

Even if you consider yourself a sensible person, as I do, why not *go for glamour*. If you are drawn to the gold, the glass, the elegance and lure of glamour, why not add more of it into your life if it makes you happy?

The kind of glamour I'm talking about is five-star: hotels with thick luxurious carpeting and a hushed atmosphere; gold and glass premium makeup counters; first-class travel; and velvety red wine in a fine-rimmed glass.

I don't travel first class however, or even premium economy. I live a normal life and place value on being a good steward of my money, so I like to find ways to add that five-star glamour into my life on a budget. I study hotel décor and see how we can borrow some of that for our home. I set up vignettes in our bedroom to mirror the luxury of the perfume counters.

Reading glossy magazines lends me that languid feeling of luxury as well. Home décor magazines give me ideas to try and colour palettes to covet; fashion magazines inspire me to have a play around in my wardrobe and see what new outfits I can make and what glamorous touches I can include (such as ropes of pearls a la Coco).

Choosing glamour encompasses all areas of my life. It inspires me to purchase the lacy cheeky panties in a pretty colour instead of the plain beige ones which are invisible under clothing. When I am considering the beige panties, I temporarily forget that there is no item of clothing I own which is sheer enough to warrant such a passion-killing piece of underwear.

So, what are all the little ways one can add glamour to their life, without breaking the budget? Here are some of my favourites:

Wear big sunglasses. They don't have to be expensive, but they can be. I would love to invest in a great pair of sunglasses because I know I look after them and will have them for years. Whenever I see someone looking alluring and chic, they are invariably wearing a striking pair of sunglasses, whether on their face or on their head.

I have also seen studies where people are rated more attractive when wearing sunglasses. Isn't it fabulous that you can become better looking *and* protect your eyesight all at the same time?

Make up your eyes. This was a whole chapter in my first *Thirty Chic Days* book and I'm still an advocate. Spending an extra five or ten minutes on your makeup is something that adds zing and fun to your day because whenever you look in the mirror you see someone that is not your everyday boring person. No, you see a glamorous smoky-eyed bombshell.

There is no cost either. You likely already own an eyeliner and eyeshadows, so why not use them? And while you're at it, pile on the mascara like there is no tomorrow. I love to keep the rest of my makeup quite sheer and pretty so that my eyes are the only focus. Natural coloured lip balm or lipstick is my go-to and I don't feel overdone.

Light candles in pretty jars. Candlelight reflecting around a room at night feels luxe and sensual, all for the price of a 40-cent tea-light. I regularly put my candle holders through the dishwasher too, ensuring they are sparkling clean and ready to glow. Charity stores are great places to pick up pretty candle glasses at low prices; that way you can keep a few in the cupboard and rotate them so you don't become bored with the same look.

Style your bed. I am quite a lazy girl and would be happy to decorate our bed with only the two pillows we sleep on. However, I want that stylish and luxe bed look more, so I add three cushions in front of our pillows. It's a small enough amount not to be a bother, and a big enough statement that our bed looks pretty every time I pass it. It is the bedroom equivalent of adding a necklace or scarf to your outfit. I change the cushion covers around every so often to keep this petite scene fresh and interesting.

Wear pretty underwear. No frumpy or practical underwear is allowed in my closet! I have decluttered the beige and the nude, the smooth and the purely comfy. Instead I now have a beautiful and inspiring collection of comfortable lacy bras which I pair with my bright lace knickers. I've worked out that I prefer butt-covering briefs to G-strings, and I keep things pretty by choosing mostly lace, and maybe cute stripes every so often (but always with a lace trim). I also have a few leopard-print pairs of knickers which are fun too.

Nothing is purely matching, *per se*, but they all go together. For example, I wear a black bra with my leopard and black knickers. I wear a peach and white lace bra with peony pink lace knickers. A navy lace bra with sheer navy/daisy embroidered knickers.

Nothing is expensive either, so I don't worry about hand-washing to preserve my investment (although I do wash all my underwear in lingerie bags; I have about a dozen of them, but it only takes a second to put one item in each bag on wash day). My bras are from K-Mart and my knickers mostly come from Victoria's Secret when they have a special offer. Putting my underwear on makes me happy every day and yes, I do feel glamorous doing that.

Use your good dishes. Maybe you won't do this every day, but it's fun to serve your meal on beautiful and special plates at least once or twice a week. Drink your tea from a pot using an antique cup and saucer. It feels so good to do this and it also elevates your dining or tea-time experience.

As with machine-washing my lingerie, I put all our dishes through the dishwasher whether they are delicate or not. A few of my items are expensive, but most are from charity stores and auctions. If I have to hand-wash something I'll probably not use it but knowing I have chosen to put everything in the dishwasher means I can regularly enjoy everything we own.

In addition, moving all our dishes to make them more easily accessible means we happily use them on an ordinary night instead of waiting for a special occasion.

Dance to *one song*. Lately I've been luring my husband into a dance while one of us is cooking dinner. This is something that sounds so twee when you read about it, but when you do it it's the most fun ever – even if both of you are terrible dancers!

You can move imperfectly and do dips by the cutlery drawer. Did you know that one song lasts a long time when you're in motion? Truly!

At the end of it you'll have reconnected with the love of your life, started the blood pumping around your body and maybe even become a little winded (I know I do). Last night I had Mambo No. 5 in my mind, so I found it on the iPod and my husband and I danced while the pasta simmered.

Look for glamorous inspiration everywhere

Living a life of glamor is mainly about removing barriers: wearing sultry makeup at home even if you're not seeing anybody (well, except for the most important people in your life: your family); choosing uplifting lingerie that will make you feel pretty; and eating your weeknight dinner off your grandmother's beautiful china or sipping your drink from a vintage glass.

When I'm watching a movie such as *Breakfast at Tiffany's* it might spark an idea such as, 'Hmm, I might start wearing a satin sleep-mask'. Or I'll see a lady in the street who looks fabulous in her high(ish) heels, so think, 'I'm going to wear my heels more' and I do, even though it might be more comfortable to wear flats. I'm not going to be silly about it and wear high heels when I have a full day on my feet, but if I'm going to the bank with my husband for a half-hour appointment, why not look and feel a touch more glamorous?

Glamour is not about spending money and being uncomfortable though. It is about choosing the luxurious option and having a small effort pay big dividends. It's about upgrading tiny areas in your life which in turn provides a sparkle to everything around them. Think about it – jeans, a crisp shirt and white sandshoes: cute. Jeans, a crisp shirt and kitten heels: Emmanuelle Alt. (Emmanuelle Alt is the editor of Vogue Paris and one of my style icons.)

It's fun to be a chic detective and pinpoint all those little ways you can elevate your style – and your life – without too much effort. No-one wants to feel like life is a big palaver, I certainly don't. I like to get the most bang for my buck and the most glamour for my exertion. Lazy glamour? I like it.

Thirty Chic Days inspirational ideas:

What glamorous touches would you like to incorporate into your life? **What lights you up?**

Just asking yourself 'what are some little ways I can **add glamour to my life** in a way that suits my style?' then trying for at least thirty answers will bring up some great ideas.

Whenever you notice a detail that whispers *glamour* to you, **note it down on your inspiration list** for future use.

Day 3
French chic and slender

In my mid-forties I started to gain weight unexpectedly. I knew I was being more 'relaxed' with my eating but eventually realized my snacking consequences were being compounded by hormonal changes.

I'd already released my book *Thirty Slim Days* with my tips and tricks for living a slender lifestyle, yet here I was increasing in size, seemingly out of my control.

I know it's a first-world problem, but I truly felt terrified that I wouldn't be able to stop the upwards slide. Was I destined for middle-aged frump and to get fatter every year towards menopause and beyond?

I spent several months in this emotional state, and it was not fun. And, of course, what makes you feel better when you are down? That's right, eating; specifically, carbs and 'fun' foods. Foods that are neither chic nor good for a healthy weight.

I knew something needed to change but looking for that change from a state of panic wasn't going to be fruitful. I needed to relax and work things out from a calm state of mind instead.

I thought, *Right, what's the one place where I can take the pressure off myself?* and it immediately came to me – my wardrobe. Many of my clothes were simply too tight and I felt bad about myself every morning when I was getting dressed.

So, I bought a few new inexpensive items to bolster my choices and replaced my bras because my boobs were getting bigger by the day. A sizeable bust runs in my family which might sound good if you haven't been 'blessed', but it's harder to hide weight gain when your bosom is massive.

Once I had a few comfortable and semi-nice looking outfits though, I could relax and start to feel better about myself. My next step was to find evidence to inspire me into healthier eating and also prove to my worried mind that middle-age spread was not a given.

Re-inspire yourself

I found the ladies who were my original inspiration all those years ago – the mythical ideal Parisian woman and some real-life chic ladies who are showing me and the rest of the world that you can be chic, slim and have a fabulous time throughout your life. By their example

I could see there was no reason to feel dumpy if I didn't want to.

I needed those real and fictitious women to inspire me into better eating habits and feel confident that one can be older and still healthy and slim.

Browsing my inspiration files with torn-out magazine articles did the trick. Dormant feelings of excitement were reignited, and this helped me to lessen my sugar intake without effort. Sugar has always been my 'go-to' to feel good ever since I was young. It is also my biggest weight contributor.

I replaced my excitement over a bar of chocolate with the promise of cultivating my own version of a chic French personal style. Instead of looking for my next sweet fix, I studied my style files for outfit ideas and grooming inspiration. I visualized daily how good I was going to look in the stylish outfits I already owned.

I looked at my style icons too. Anyone can look good when youth is on their side; but it's the ladies who are older than me that I wanted to search out: women such as Emmanuelle Alt (51), Carine Roitfeld (63) and Kristin Scott Thomas (58). These ladies are all slender and healthy looking, as well as having a personal style that is ageless and timeless. They are very much 'younger than their age'.

Studying them showed me that middle-age frump was optional, not compulsory; a choice, not a given. I also took note of what they wore when I liked the way they looked. Perhaps there were some minor style additions I could take on board while I trimmed down my weight.

One of my style tweaks was to wear more structured items, such as an ironed cotton shirt with the sleeves rolled up instead of a knit top. Men always look so much more pulled together in a crisp shirt than a tee-shirt, so I took that inspiration for myself. I also noted that tailored lines were more flattering to a not-so-perfect figure.

Some of my shirts were too tight across the bust, but some of my looser cut ones were fine. I was pleased to add another few items to my temporary wardrobe.

Take the focus off food

Once I had put together a capsule collection, I enjoyed inspiring myself daily with Internet style searches, viewings of chic French movies such as *Madame* and brainstorming inspiration in my journal. As a result, eating became less fretful.

I didn't crave carby breakfasts and lunches, and was happy to choose my fruit, yoghurt and raw nuts or a smoothie packed with goodness. I was happy not to bring any sugary treat foods into the house.

I also forgave myself when I didn't eat perfectly – I had potato chips a few times each week and a small sweet treat after lunch. There are some sweet bites that don't cause me to go nuts and eat the whole packet, such as very dark chocolate – 90% cacao is my favourite.

I was slimming down the way I wanted to live my life forever, and I knew I could not be a flawless eater for decades on end. Life is not a controlled laboratory environment, rather it's messy and imperfect. Falling apart and going for broke was how I used to deal with 'breaking my diet'. *But that was the old me,* I'd tell myself, *I am different now.*

And so I went on – inspiring myself to enjoy fashion and style, and therefore eat better. I didn't follow a formal plan, simply trusted that I'd know best what to eat or not eat.

There are other factors too: how we look and feel isn't only indicative of what we've been eating and drinking. It reflects how we have been sleeping, whether we are putting ourselves under stress or not, and how much we have been moving – so many factors.

All the scientific stuff is too boring to think about for me. All I need to know is that I must work on feeling good by:

- Inspiring myself with beautiful possibility.
- Getting excited about creating colourful and delicious meals with real ingredients.
- Enjoy doing my hair and makeup each day – my motto is quick and simple, and I do it early so I can feel good the whole day long.
- Having blissfully early nights with a good book.

- Smiling a lot and appreciating all the goodness I already have in my life.

- Have fun wearing as many different items in my closet as I can and accessorising even at home.

- Anticipate and visualize wearing outfits that I haven't worn for a long time – this is one of my favourite ways to drift off to sleep at night, running a little movie in my head of me getting dressed in something fabulous (whether it's casual or dressed up) and travelling or going out for a drink at a hot new bar. It's fun to do, I never have trouble nodding off plus it has a good future outcome because I am implanting that vision into my mind.

- Keep reminding myself 'this is the new me', 'this is my new normal' and not getting sucked back into old stories and excuses.

- Journaling scenarios to keep my spirits above reality and inspiring myself into loftier thoughts. 'Writing my own happy ending' in other words.

May I offer to you that creating your own inspiration is a far more fun option than starting a new diet?

Diets are insidious in that they lure you in with the promise of an easy and permanent fix, but they are anything but. After a few weeks or even a matter of days when you're bored with how restrictive the plan is, you feel like you've failed again and go on an almighty blow-out. Sometimes I've lasted several months on a strict diet, but they all end the same way – in tears!

We *know* what to eat, we *know* what is beneficial and what is not. Half the time I think I am rebelling against my own wishes when I eat something with many calories and zero nutrition. But by letting the strictness go, there is no rebellion needed. How soothing is that?

If you are ready to try a new approach, one that is radically against the grain of any diet wisdom, why not *inspire yourself instead*?

Thirty Chic Days inspirational ideas:

Write your reality into being. Next time you are feeling down and like you are destined to live in a body that is always going to weigh more than you'd like, grab your journal.

This is where inspiration starts. You can feel free to write down things that inspire you. It is your secret garden where you can really be yourself. Do not dismiss any idea as too tiny or shallow; I often find these are the thoughts that spark the best actions.

Ten ideas. I love to write down lists of ideas that excite me (I try for ten each day). It could be a meal idea, an outfit I've seen on television, a style icon I've been channelling lately or a movie I want to preserve by remembering its name and a few words to describe the feeling of it.

I usually start off my daily list of ten with the question 'What feels exciting to me right now?'

Questions. I also love to journal answers to enticing questions. Ten is quick and easy, but twenty is great if you are in the mood and want to spend a little more time journaling.

Little sparkly gems of ideas and thoughts come from this practice, and doing it regularly keeps your mind high in the sky where possibility is endless, instead of in the pantry looking for a snack.

Here are a few of my favourites to start you off.

What is my ideal vision for my personal style?

If I had an idealized style, what would it reference?

What kind of daily things would I love to do in my perfect life?

Why do I want to live like this?

What are ten outfits from my wardrobe that I know would look amazing on the new me?

What are ten projects that I'd love to complete this year?

Who are my current style icons and why do I admire them?

What are ten chic lunch ideas that are yummy, easy and healthy?

How can I inspire myself with my closet?

Just to give you an idea, here is how I answered that last journal question:

1. Take outfit photos laid out on the carpet so I can be inspired to wear those outfits soon

2. Go through my out-of-season clothing bins and see what I've got

3. Start taking daily outfit photos again

4. Inspire myself by browsing my skinny clothes and imagining how good they will look

5. Look at scarf tying ideas and wear my scarves more

6. Create my ideal 'French girl' capsule wardrobe

7. Identify my current favourite colour palette

8. Iron all my shirts and enjoy wearing them

9. Get all the clothes that fit me well right now and wear them, even if they are a bit too fancy for every day

10. Be inspired to declutter and reorganize my closet by viewing ladies with minimal wardrobes online

And, one of my 10 ideas lists:

1. Quit the gym if I want to
2. Walk every day
3. Drink lots of lovely water
4. Wear my retainers at night
5. Use my Clarisonic brush in the evening
6. Add to my charity donation box in the car
7. Choose a daily mantra each morning to remember what I want
8. Love my life every day
9. Say thank you a lot
10. Be happy, enjoy life, play with my husband and be fun

I hope this chapter has inspired you to be light and playful yourself and know that your weight is not a serious matter. It's just your body, and you can be different if you want to. Happy inspiration, chic friend!

Day 4
Live a five-star life

I am happiest when living my simple and beautiful life at home, and I'm also a thrifty and practical person. However... I love to add sparkly highlights to my everyday life with the thoughts of living a jet set, luxurious five-star life of glamour and travel.

Being a homebody and an introvert, it's often more fun for me to have this as my frame of mind and let it brighten the colours of my daily living than to pursue that five-star vacation for real. I think this is a recurring theme for me – daydreaming of something is often better than the reality!

Of course, I love going on holiday, but why spend the in-between times waiting and wishing for your next trip? I can look forward to our next vacation, whenever that might be, but in the meantime I do my best to make every single day of my life enjoyable, and with luxurious touches as well.

Only take notice of five-star reviews

I love to read Amazon reviews of books I want to read (or have already read), but mostly I'll only read the five-star reviews. I realized I was doing this by accident, and then carried on.

It happened when I visited a book I'd read and loved. For some reason I clicked on the one-star reviews and found that I started taking on all the terrible opinions of the book and all the things that were wrong with it.

These reviews coloured the book for me and I couldn't 'unhear' their opinions. It's human nature that people love to complain, but really, who wants to hear others' fault-finding? Surely there's enough negativity in life without going out looking for more?

I found the opposite to be true when I read five-star reviews exclusively. These reviewers pick out excellent points I may not have considered before; they might share a list of their highlights from the book and in the case of non-fiction titles, can sometimes helpfully summarize the main points.

Often the five-star reviews themselves are highly motivating and I find myself buoyed by them because they have been written by happy, effervescent people who are sharing their joy. Just like when you come across someone positive in real life, they make you feel good and like anything is possible.

In addition, reading five-star reviews gives me a new appreciation for a book that I have already read and enjoyed, and I'll often end up re-reading it and gaining even more pleasure from it. I am a great fan of re-reading favourite books, even though it seems a terrible waste of time because there are so many books I want to read. It's like a mental comfort blanket since you know what's coming up. And when it's a favourite non-fiction book, don't you find you receive new messages from it with each read? I certainly do.

Before I decided that I will only read the good reviews and not the bad, seeing many different opinions on the same book reminded me that we all look at what's in front of us in diverse ways – it goes along with the saying, 'one man's trash is another man's treasure'. But why wallow in the trash when you can glory in the treasure?

In the past I've clicked through to the profile of a one-star book reviewer if their review seems quite mean, and I'll see that they give moany negative reviews to *everything*. This goes to show that they'll likely never be happy with anything they've ordered, be it a book, a pair of stretch leggings or a cheese grater. They look for things to complain about and they'll always find them.

From this experience I thought to myself: *Why not choose to look for the five-star experiences in your life instead of the one-stars, Fiona? You'll find both because both exist, but which would make you happier?*

Give your life five-star reviews

My five-star review experiment gave me the idea to only rate things in my life as five-star as well. After all, why not? Why not give five-star reviews for anything I do in my life? I don't want a one-star life! And if I only focus on the good, it means I am constantly upgrading which can only lead to a fabulous future.

Instead of thinking to myself, 'Why did I stay up so late last night and now I've slept in wasting my Sunday morning?', I can change it to, 'Way to go enjoying that movie. Make the most of a rare Sunday sleep-in. Life is for the living! A five-star weekend!'

Instead of looking at a meal I cooked and thinking, 'I could have used a bit more seasoning' I'll tell myself, 'Five stars! Look at the perfect crispness of the steamed asparagus!' and, 'How delicious is that roast potato?'

And to *receive* five-star reviews with pleasure as well: 'Why thank you, yes, it was a delicious meal!' rather than, 'Oh it was okay, the gravy was a bit thin though, don't you think?' Go on, admit that you've deflected compliments in the past like I have. Instead, why not give both the compliment-giver and yourself the gift of receiving thoughtful words graciously.

Living your five-star life

What I love most about my five-star life is that it also feels like I am calling it five-star in the luxury hotel kind of way. I am inspired to keep my home tidy and clutter-free, because shoes by the sofa and a pile of old newspapers is *not* five-star.

Just having the phrase 'five-star' in mind reminds me of my desire to live in a luxurious yet simple way. This mindset makes the everyday feel special. Looking for the five-starness in everything I do helps me always look on the bright side and look for the best in every situation too.

I'm sure any of us could easily rate something as one-star or five-stars depending on what part of it we were looking at, whether it's a book, our home or how well we are doing at work.

I'm reminded of this in different situations. One example is a group of us going out for dinner. I'd think to myself, 'what a lovely ambience this restaurant has, I feel so cool and stylish being here' when one of my dining companions might point out someone badly dressed and pop my gold-tinted thought bubble.

I have been that picky never-happy person in the past too, so please don't think I am Little Miss Perfect radiating sunshine wherever she goes. I talk about this in my book *Thirty Chic Days*, in *Day 11: Adopt a low-drama way of being*. After realizing that my critical hyper-focus was not making me happy but in fact the complete opposite, I worked on turning my mind around to become more tolerant, accepting and content.

My husband has a friend who is financially very successful. He's built big businesses, travelled a lot and has a beautiful wife and children. And, he is the most ridiculously positive person you've ever met. Comically so, and has been known to exclaim 'I love life! Life is excellent!' Everything is wonderful, nothing's ever a problem and my husband jokingly said that no-one in their right mind would take a restaurant recommendation from him because even if they served him up an old shoe he'd rave about the place. He would find something to praise enthusiastically and not notice anything bad.

My husband has been friends with this fellow since he was five years old, and said he's always been that way. One day I decided to borrow his over-the-top *joie de vivre* and see if it couldn't benefit me too. And do you know what, it has. I'm not perfect at it and can still slip into my old complainy ways, but most of the time I rave about service, focus on the good things in my experience and talk people up.

I'll never be as crazily enthusiastic as he is, because my own demeanour is quite quiet, but this small change has been a fun one to embrace and has definitely helped my luck factor. I look around at how different my life is from even five years ago and can't help but smile. I feel so lucky!

This change did not come naturally to me since I've been cynical and looking for small details to correct for most of my life, so I built it up slowly. The last thing I want to be is inauthentic, and I couldn't be anyway. So I started by giving five-star reviews to everything I experience and day-by-day this has led to me creating my own five-star life.

Treat yourself like a VIP

Part of the five-star life is feeling like a Very Important Person, and it's not only about spending money either. In my world something as simple as having cleanliness around me makes me feel like a VIP. An example is the cozy white robe that I put on every morning while I write, sipping on my special giant 'morning mug' of hot tea. Washing it regularly feels good and doesn't take any more effort than throwing it in with a load of towels.

This may sound basic, but I didn't always wash my fluffy robe as frequently because it was a bulky item and would fill up the machine, and I reasoned that I only wore it for an hour or so each day. But when I thought about the robes at a five-star hotel, they are always pristinely white and fluffy and make me feel like a million dollars when I wrap myself up in them.

Little details like this are easy and inexpensive to recreate at home and all add to that VIP five-star feeling. Other areas that make me feel 'rich' are:

- **Crisply ironed shirts** lined up in my closet ready to wear. I used to hate ironing and would do anything to avoid it, even though I love the look and feel of a freshly pressed cotton or linen shirt on myself. I would hang my shirts up wrinkled, and iron them as I wore them. One day something clicked and now I love to iron my shirts straight from the line – even better if they are still slightly damp because this makes the job even easier and with a better result.

- Having one or two **glossy picture books** on the coffee table and giving myself time to flick through them (I rotate them from my bookshelf so they always seem fresh to my eyes, even though I bought them years ago).

- **Running the dishwasher** when it's almost full, rather than having every nook and cranny filled. It's not such an ordeal to unload and feels like we are on holiday in a serviced apartment when we'd run the dishwasher each night. Yes, I am thrifty and quite green as well, but the levels I'd go to were getting ridiculous waiting for *just one more meal* to turn the dishwasher on.

Remember what inspires you

One thing that effortlessly motivates me to make positive changes towards my five-star life is my love affair with Paris and the South of France. Any little reminder helps rekindle my initial excitement around the world of French Chic and remember that I desire to be the chicest and best version of myself.

Enjoying ten minutes browsing through one of my big picture books such as Vicki Archer's 'My French Life' is a fabulous boost to my happiness.

Browsing a fancy Parisian hotel online and viewing the gallery of photos does too. I love to stage my living areas and bedroom regularly (sometimes daily) by removing all the tiny items of clutter and taking care of the details such as plumping cushions and straightening magazines, just like they would in a five-star hotel.

This in turn spills over into eating better, dressing with panache more often and feeling more confident when I'm out. It's one big beautiful chain reaction.

Thirty Chic Days inspirational ideas:

- Firstly, decide that you are going to live a five-star lifestyle if this concept appeals to you.

- Then, make incremental upgrades over time – growing gradually into your new way of being feels comfortable and is more sustainable.

- Look for good quality when you come to replace something – this won't necessarily be the most expensive option either.

- Elevate how your surroundings feel by using things up, clearing out and decluttering. Ask yourself, 'Does this item belong in my five-star life?'

- When you look into your closet and feel uninspired, think to yourself, 'What pieces feel worthy of my five-star life?' or 'How can I create a five-star wardrobe?'

- Wear something that is 'too good' for everyday use and enjoy the compliments you receive. You will likely hold yourself more elegantly and take different actions too. I love to mix a slightly dressier top with jeans; add to this a pair of heels and you'll feel like a celebrity heading out to the latest nightspot. For me, it is a combo that never fails.

- Make a promise to yourself that you are going to be the most annoyingly passionate and positive person you know, starting today!

Day 5
Get your sexy back

As I write this I am forty-seven. You may be younger, older or the same age as me. What I can tell you is that when you are forty-seven, frumpiness sneaks in the side door when you are not looking. And without you even realizing has you caring less about what you eat, starts putting frumpy clothes in your closet and decides that you are going to wear practical full briefs instead of lacy panties... Perhaps she has been to your house too?

And now that I think about it, frumpiness isn't just because of age; I remember having times when I felt and looked frumpy in my twenties and thirties as well. Frump is not ageist, sadly, so we must be ever vigilant!

I happened to be browsing the Victoria's Secret website and found myself feeling so envious of all those happy-looking slender women, dancing around in their cute sleepshirts, zippy athletic-ware and colourful lingerie.

I felt a bit dumpy in myself, not because of my physical shape, although I'd happily lose a few pounds; no, it was more my state of mind that was stuck. I felt unmotivated, dowdy and heavy of spirit.

I thought that ordering some new underwear online would help alleviate that, but then I skipped forward in my mind to receiving my Victoria's Secret parcel and seeing that the pieces I ordered would *not* look the same on me as the pictures on the website.

It's not that I am unhappy with my body, I'm just realistic. I look different to those young, genetically gifted models who aren't allowed to eat much. It's their job to look good in underwear and they got the job because of that.

Instead I tried a different approach and spent the next ten minutes quickly brainstorming what it was about those ladies that I was transfixed by.

In creating this list, I inspired myself to not just buy the lacy panties (which I did), but embody the kind of person I desired to be whether I shopped on this website or not. I inhabited the mindset by noting down everything I admired about the images they were portraying and how I could create that same feeling for myself. Here is what I came up with.

My Victoria's Secret Life:

Sexy, playful and fun

Wholesome and healthy
Flirty panties and happy smiles
Plaid pyjama pants and a long-sleeve T
Sexy bra and knickers with a kimono gown
Curled up in leggings and a cozy top sipping coffee from a big mug
Angels and bombshells
Deliciously scented
Every man's dream
The ideal girlfriend
Making the most of your looks
Cute and sporty
Athletic and youthful
Sultry, sexy and sensual
Tanned and toned
Fresh and new

Since creating this inspiration for myself I have felt more inspired to *be* that lady – in my own way – rather than passively taking in images and placing orders online. Instead of feeling down on myself because I don't look exactly like them, I can be inspired to be *my* best self by acting as if.

I have been using my NutriBullet to make a **quick, extremely healthy and delicious** lunch when at home by myself, because that's what *she* would do.

I decluttered underwear in preparation for receiving my seven new pairs of pretty knickers, and now

everything in my lingerie drawer makes me feel good. Streamlining my underwear drawer of anything worn-out or frumpy made me feel fresh and new, and I had plenty of room for my lacy Victoria's Secret panties when they arrived.

I am normally quite a thrifty person, but I even got rid of a few pairs that were technically still okay because I didn't feel like my most desirable self while wearing them. They weren't new but they weren't old either. Their crime was that they had the energy of someone middle-aged who had given up, and I decided that was *not* the energy I wanted to be surrounded by!

I started dressing in clothes at home that made me feel **cute, playful and attractive**. Sure, they may still have been jeans and tee-shirts, but the jeans were fitted stretch fabric, and the tee-shirts were in flattering feminine colours and shapes (both my current jeans and tee-shirts are from Kmart, so it's not like they cost a lot either).

Maybe you are someone who instinctively gravitates towards sexiness, whether it's your culture or just your natural state of being. Lucky you. For me, even in my teens and twenties I veered more towards classic/conservative/staid.

I always wanted to look nice, but it was far easier to skip that for another day and slip into something more comfortable (which is the opposite in real life than when they say it in the movies).

By cleaning out my closet of anything that could remotely be considered frumpy, I couldn't wear those pieces because they weren't there anymore. It's the same concept as not keeping your nemesis treat foods in the house, so you don't end up eating them.

I also started creating more direction to follow, by taking my inspiration notes at the beginning of this chapter and asking myself questions such as:

How can I feel more sexy, playful and fun?

How can I make the most of my looks?

How can I feel athletic and youthful?

What could I do that would feel fresh and new?

Action steps I came up for myself included:

Taking my neighbour's poodle Teddy for a walk and jogging some of the time too. (This was before we had adopted our own dogs). Teddy is an exuberant three-year old medium-sized poodle and he loves to run. Normally I'd let him tug on the leash as I walked, but when I started running alongside him it felt joyous and playful. I didn't run the entire way, that would have just about killed me, so I alternated **walking and jogging** as he stopped and started.

Running with Teddy made me feel **athletic and youthful**, but I also helped this along by buying some new workout clothes. I hadn't bought any for a long time – years in fact. Some of my tee-shirts were worn out – there were little and not-so-little holes under the arms for goodness sake – and I only had two pairs of capri-length leggings, so both were often in the wash at the same time.

I bought myself four new tops and three new pairs of leggings from the sports section at, again, Kmart (these items are surprisingly nice and cost only $8 and $12 each respectively), so I now have cute and practical clothes ready to go.

I started **wearing a tiny amount of makeup every day** instead of just sometimes. It takes less than ten minutes and I feel good all day. It only takes an extra five minutes to wash it off at night, making a total daily investment of fifteen-minutes.

To help with this, I streamlined my makeup tray into a small core of items that I could use every morning. I cleaned my makeup brushes and cases, and everything felt fresh and new.

Being that woman now

In my head I felt fresh and new too, from all these little actions I was taking – and the new way I was thinking. Now when I look at my original inspiration list I know I am becoming that woman I admire. She feels light of spirit and happy within herself. She smiles genuinely and knows that even if she doesn't have a perfect figure, she is loving and accepting of herself and will live her life happily. She chooses to give love to her health and wellbeing too.

She focuses on all the goodness she can add into her day – moving in a fun way, keeping hydrated, eating simple home-cooked meals and finding pleasure in many different ways, not just with food. She reads books she loves and spends time with family and friends. She keeps her home tidy and clean because a pleasing environment lifts her up.

She chooses not to be self-conscious about her self-perceived flaws, and instead pours joy into whomever she is socializing with. She looks at them with loving eyes and is fully focused on what they are saying. When she speaks, only positive words come from her mouth and they are on interesting topics. She forgets all about her prior nervousness and fully enjoys the occasion.

This is how to live life, she realizes. Not by feeling isolated and stuck with only her unhelpful comfortable habits to keep her company, but by embracing that dreamy idealized version of how she wishes to be.

Thirty Chic Days inspirational ideas:

Create your own inspiration to get *your* sexy back. Firstly, what kind of sexy do you desire? Is it deeply sensual? Playful and fun? Cool and insouciant? Brainstorm a list of ways you'd like to be; you know, in your ideal world. *The movie you.* Personally, I love to be inspired by movies I have seen.

Then, look at all the ways you can **be that person** from the outside-in (with the actions you take) and the inside-out (with the thoughts you think). Ask yourself what that version of yourself would do, and what her mindset would look like?

Write down everything you can think of, even the seemingly inconsequential specifics. I find for me that those tiny details which might seem silly to others effortlessly propel my motivation. They give flight to my elevated way of being, and they are easy to fit into my life right now. They are my secret little gems, sparkling brightly and lighting my way.

Aim to bring these small changes into your day and read through your inspiration list often. Picture yourself living your fabulous life as *her*. Breathe in that feeling of hope, wonder and excitement.

This is how I got my sexy back when I found it had slipped... lost somewhere on the side of the road in Frumpyville. But I don't live there anymore, and you don't have to either if you don't want to.

Day 6

Be your own chic mentor

Think about the last time you visited the home of someone stylish. If you're anything like me, you will have been observing how they live – looking around to see their décor, books on the shelves, noticing what they serve for dinner or afternoon tea, and peeking at their perfumes when you visit the bathroom. (Go on, I know you do!).

Or perhaps you follow your favourite celebrities on Instagram and live for the days when they post snippets of their lives, personal style secrets and photos of their home interior.

I love to observe stylish ladies (and sometimes men) because it gives me ideas and also the strength to live my own life of elegance and refinement. Seeing how others hold high standards for themselves helps me remember that it's okay to want to live with flair and panache and have that high standard for myself as well.

Sometimes those chic sightings are thin on the ground though. Life can seem hum-drum and you're more drawn to snack foods and junky television than styling your closet and going for a walk.

Those personally are the times when I could use a shot in the arm – a shot of chic!

If you've ever thought: 'I wish there were examples of ladies around me – not just in movies or magazines – that were living an amazing, quality life', I have an idea for you. *Be that role model you wish you had. Invent her for yourself.*

Write down all the things that your ideal role model would be, do and have, and then claim that for your own reality.

For me, my ideal role model is brave - embracing changes such as new technology, not fearing the future, becoming better and better over time and having fun in her everyday.

She loves how she's chosen to live her life, not having just gone along with what everyone else does or what her friends and family think would be best for her.

She has actively gone out and chosen exactly how she desires to spend her days, highlighting the fact that she wants a life of ease and simplicity. She chooses how she wants to work and earn an income, how she looks, how she spends her money, and what and who she surrounds herself with.

She loves herself at every stage of her life. She plays up her physical strengths and forgets about her self-professed 'flaws'. She excels in focusing on her positive attributes.

She loves creating outfits that reflect her desired personal style. She feels youthful and sexy, no matter her age. She knows that sensuality and a youthful outlook are a state of mind, not numerical fact.

By brainstorming all the sorts of attributes I wish to continue cultivating in my life, I feel more inspired than ever and it's easy to elevate my standards again, effortless in fact.

By doing an exercise such as this for yourself, you are tapping into your inner wisdom and generating feelings of excitement about what's to come, at the same time as enjoying yourself right now.

Can you see how this way of thinking would naturally lead you to act in a way that is more conducive to living a happy, healthy and enjoyable life? I can, and I've proved it to myself over and over.

Having this broad picture of how you wish to be then leads you into all the delightful little details you could infuse into your day – details that remind you of your high standards. I then turn all those details into affirmations to inspire myself...

I dress with care each day, even if I'm 'just at home'
I have a minimum of makeup that I choose to wear daily
I enjoy adorning myself with my everyday jewellery and occasionally costume jewellery
I use my pretty china and wash it in the dishwasher
I wear lacy bras and knickers every day
I have decluttered my entire closet of anything remotely frumpy
I plant red geraniums in terracotta pots on the patio
I enjoy a glass of wine before dinner
I sip water all day long and love feeling hydrated
I make time to read every day
I go to bed at a reasonable hour
I have at-home facial masks once or twice a week
I make the effort to go to local events when they appeal
I invite friends around for coffee or dinner
I regularly organize and declutter my home: kitchen, closet, office, computer, books and magazines
I take care to enjoy the pretty details such as flicking through a glossy picture book, lighting a scented candle or writing in a new notebook
I plan for meals and prepare ingredients ahead of time
I watch movies that inspire me
I browse my style files often
I keep in touch with family and friends by phone or email, just to say 'Hi'
I journal new ideas for myself regularly

I take the time to dream and plan
I let myself enjoy my life

It is wonderful to be inspired by others, but it's far more satisfying to be inspired by your own thoughts, because everything you do will then be exquisitely fashioned to your taste. Being your own chic mentor can only lead to great things, and you will enjoy yourself so much along the way that you will only periodically look around for external motivation. It's a beautiful upwards spiral where you become happier and more fulfilled over time.

Spreading happiness

Even when life happens, because it does to all of us, you will be better able to cope with setbacks. Brainstorming your own inspirational ideas might sound shallow and a 'nice to have' but not necessary; I believe it is anything but. By having a life that makes you happy every day you will naturally radiate a sunnier disposition than if you simply plodded along listening to the news, talking about reality television and complaining alongside your co-workers.

This positive way of being will not only elevate your happiness level, but it can't help but spread sunshine to those around you without you even realizing it. You will inspire others with how you live your life and the ripples will spread far.

When you appreciate the life you have and make the most of it regardless of whether external circumstances are perfect, you really are living the life of your dreams. Because even if you won the lottery and never had money worries ever again, there would still be things in your life that were bothersome.

There will probably never be a time for any of us that we could rightfully say, 'I have no concerns right now' so we are letting our life drip away day by day if we are waiting for that time. Rather than putting your enjoyment on hold until life is 'under control', love it now, imperfect circumstances, non-thin thighs, annoying boss and all. Love all of it and decide that you are exactly where you are meant to be.

Even now when I have my dream lifestyle working from home writing books, there are still days I can feel as if life is a drag, and it's all because I am not cultivating my inner landscape. On a down day I might look back at my earlier life in my teens, twenties and thirties and think 'life was so much fun back then'.

But if I *really* remember correctly, sure I did have a lot of fun (which I made myself) but I was always thinking of this beautiful future when I could be at home full-time. When I was catching the bus to work on a rainy day I'd think to myself, '*Oh, imagine not having to leave the house on a day like this. I could enjoy my home and potter around. It would be wonderful.*'

I am such a homebody and adore being a happy homemaker that it was a dream for me to spend the entire day at home if I wanted to – and now I can do that. So why was I glorifying the past when I now have everything I've ever wanted?

These nostalgic thoughts threatening to overshadow my present day proved to me that it doesn't really matter – within reason – your circumstances, you can make the most of them and cultivate your most expansive life.

Gosh, when I've switched my mindset around again (say, if I've gone off the boil and start thinking life is mundane and what's the point of doing those little feminine touches) it's as if a light has been switched on and everything is glittering and hopeful and shimmering again.

Isn't it funny how we constantly have to re-remember sometimes?

By being a chic mentor to ourselves and creating our own inspiration, we can be reminded of our wishes more often. We won't let ourselves get to that drudging state where we don't care so much about what we wear or go for that stodgy food that we don't particularly care for but eat anyway.

When we are lifting ourselves up through our own self-coaching, we effortlessly take the better path and enjoy doing so. We can't imagine wanting to eat junky food or flomp around in pyjamas all day. No, we're springing out of bed in the morning to prepare a delicious fresh breakfast before choosing how we want to present ourselves to the world. Suddenly everything is clear and it's as if the sun has just come out.

Thirty Chic Days inspirational ideas:

Create a big picture that is compelling. Ask yourself what you want your life to look and feel like as you go forward. Paint with broad strokes and dream about the kind of person you want to become. How does *she* ideally spend her day?

Craft details of that picture into your everyday right now. Take the time to curate a big list of tiny actions that you would enjoy infusing into your life. In every idea there will be something that calls to you, or you would never have thought it up.

Choose one or two and do them today. On your list, what are one or two examples that look easy and fun? Can you try some of them right now? I promise you that by doing this you will instantly elevate yourself from the hum-drum of daily life and remember once again that your days are precious and worthy of your full attention.

An example of this for me are red geraniums as mentioned earlier in this chapter. Ever since I first read a glossy coffee table book about living in Provence and the South of France (in the 1980s! a long time ago!), I have imagined my home having a pot or two of red geraniums outside. That detail is one that anchors a feeling of happiness and gallic *joie de vivre* for me.

Every so often I grew geraniums in my garden but hadn't for a while. Recently my husband and I visited a local vineyard for a day outing where we picked grapes and had lunch with other wine enthusiasts. It was a glorious experience. Walking to the vines with our group of twenty or so people, we passed a planter massed with red geraniums. They spoke to me instantly.

A few days later I spent less than $20 for a couple of trays of geranium plants and some outdoor potting mix to fill the terracotta pots I had sitting empty in our garage. As I type this they are sitting outside being watered by the rain and I know they will create a beautiful vignette which will make me feel joyful every day for a long time.

This is the power of including little details of your dream life into your everyday, and I hope you take the time to become a chic mentor to yourself. Your happiness and the happiness of those around you is worth it.

Day 7
Find your dream life filter

I belonged to an online forum many years ago which was full of Francophile ladies all talking about how they were making their lives more *French* and *chic*.

It was a wonderful forum and the first time I saw that there were other ladies out there like me. Ladies who desired to live a beautiful life of their own design; who weren't prepared to put up with mediocrity; who were inspired to make their own life wonderful right now by sprinkling Euro-magic fairy dust over everything.

One of the forum participants – the ever-inspiring Janice from *The Vivienne Files* blog – was preparing to partake in long-term travel through Europe. Part of that trip meant her living on a French barge boat for a length of time. Hence, the 'barge filter' was born. In the leadup to her going away (and I'm sure the trip took a long time to plan and pay for), everything she bought had to be able to move to a new country and go on the barge with her.

I've always remembered the barge filter, firstly because she referenced it often, and also because it struck a chord with me. It would make everything so easy with a definiteness of purpose like that, whether you were decluttering or deciding if you wanted to purchase something in the first place. Decisions would suddenly become clear cut.

My 'life change' filter

Moving to a new house, as we did this year – and not only moving house but moving to a region six hours drive away – was the perfect filter to stop many purchases for my husband and I as well. Our lifestyle change had been in the planning for at least two years, so everything had to pass through our 'house move' filter. I'm sure you've found the same when moving to a different home.

We put an embargo on new purchases and when we did need something, it had to pass the house move test. We slept on a creaky old bed because we were going to buy a new bed when we moved. We bought no new furniture except for an essential pair of sofas (ours were literally falling to pieces under us), because when we found our new home we'd know better what furniture was needed.

Once settled into our new home, we started replacing items. We were lucky enough to get in touch with a local interior designer when we ordered a second pair of sofas through her (we inherited two living areas with our new home), and *she got our style*. She came around to our house and helped us choose paint colours for our living areas and master bedroom and gave us tips on how to achieve the style we desired.

We didn't have a name for how we wanted our home to look, so to help show her what we loved I turned to my style files where I'd ripped out magazine pages for years. I went through the stack and pulled my favourites – looks that I still loved. Then, I got my husband to go through my favourites and choose *his* favourites, thus refining the vision further and reflecting both our tastes. (It's lucky that we have a similar sensibility with what we like; I imagine how hard it would be if we had opposing wishes.)

With this bundle of 20-30 pages, we spread them out on our dining table, ready for her to view. It was fun to watch her pick out details from the pictures and hear how we could incorporate them into our new-to-us home.

The Ralph Filter

Going through my stash of home style images, I found a few Ralph Lauren Home advertisements I'd torn out. They said to me, *This! This is our look!* And the other non-Ralph images blended in to give us a look of Ralph

Lauren, so I decided that our style was to be called 'Ralph Lauren (on a budget): English country with a dash of French chateau'.

More than anything perhaps, it's the philosophy of Ralph Lauren that I love, and we wanted to embrace the feeling of that. Yes, I looked at the details of the images to see how I could recreate some looks, but I also wanted to absorb the ambience of those advertisements and then filter the feeling through my own sensibility. It was...

The patina of pre-lived furniture

Layering items over time to create a rich tapestry of textures and colours

The combination of refined English country style with a touch of glamour, and in my case, a touch of down-to-earth New Zealandness

Choosing style over fashion

Appreciating utility items

Owning pieces that get better with age

Choosing quality items made from honest materials

Mixing second-hand with new

Combining good taste, a sultry mood, elegance, and easy luxury

Keeping a sense of style in every part of our life

Ralph reminds me not to be complacent with my surroundings. To not choose the first bedside table I see because I'm sick of the cheapies I've lived with for too long now. I trusted that the perfect pair would come along, and they did.

To shortcut the decision-making process when furnishing my house – gosh, furnishing my life! – I'd ask myself 'Would Ralph choose this?' I am sure Ralph is a discerning character and would not settle for second-best. I am like that too, or I was.

Then... life got busy. It was easier to settle. But do you know what happens when you settle over and over? You end up with a life full of items, experiences and people that you don't absolutely love. And that's when you think, 'Meh'.

I am lucky enough that my first husband left me; yes, he decluttered himself! It wasn't that he was a bad person and I know I'm not, but by staying in that relationship we would have been settling. I am always in favour of people working things out and when I hear of people separating I think, 'Why? Couldn't you talk about it?' But looking back at my own marriage it was so easy to see that we were better to set ourselves free.

That's what my Ralph Lauren filter is about. Being discerning enough to know when something is not good enough for you. And I don't apply it to my relationships, just so you know, but it's proving great for not only our home style, but my personal style as well. Everything I do at the moment is passing through my Ralph filter:

Furniture we are choosing

Items I am decluttering

When I am being lazy with my outfits

Ralph's unwavering commitment to personal style in every part of his life helps inspire me to elevate my surroundings and personal style a little bit at a time, within my budget and also within my own personal style. I am not going to start wearing polo shirts because preppy is not my thing, but I *am* going to take the romance and drama from his way of looking at the world and see how I can dress in a way that reflects *my* inner world.

I'm going to wear the crisp shirt and jeans with sheer red lipstick and ballet flats to channel my inner Parisienne. I'm going to wear a big looped scarf and hair a bit mussed like the French fashion girls on Instagram.

I'm going to build my personal style to reflect the feeling of elegance, chic and love of denim that is inside me. I'm going to hunt out camel-coloured pieces within my budget because I love the luxe look of caramel tones with tan leather and tortoiseshell accessories yet have never recreated it for myself.

Once you've found your dream filter, using it doesn't require spending lots of money. In fact, it helps me not to spend money because the feeling of my Ralph filter is to use what you have, go for old, make do and mend etc.

And when you have to buy something anyway, whether it's a new winter jersey or a dining table because yours is tiny, old and cheap (or at least ours was), why not have it be the best you can find at that time and for what you are prepared to spend?

I know it's easy to feel worn down and tired and think. 'Can't someone make this easy for me?' This is how I felt about finding antique or second-hand furniture to build our home décor look on a budget. Our interior designer told us we'd get a higher quality item for much less – at least half – than we'd pay in a furniture store if we bought second-hand. 'But it's so much bother...' I thought to myself.

Now I am thinking about it another way and it's thanks to my Ralph filter. Ralph wouldn't go into a big-box store and choose over-priced faux wood furniture that won't last five years. No, he'd probably find his in a barn at an estate sale. Or he did when he was younger and broker as I have read in books about him. When he was setting up his first shop-in-shop at Bloomingdales in New York City, he and the store fit-out designer furnished his concession with second-hand finds to create the look he was after at a price he could afford.

That's what I am going for. That's my Ralph filter. And by doing so, the look that evolves over time will be far more luxurious than a bought-in-one-day matching set. As easy as that would be, I want more. Having

Ralph as my inspiration helped me feel excited by the hunt. And as our interior designer friend said to me in a wise and gentle tone when I told her of a dining suite I'd seen in a store: 'You can do better than that'.

Thirty Chic Days inspirational idea:

Choose your filter. What about you? Does this chapter suggest someone who inspires you to elevate your personal standards?

You've read about my home décor filter, but what about other areas of your life? For me, I could also have filters such as my ideal Parisian girl for my wardrobe, grooming and how I eat and drink. Or Aerin Lauder when I desire to be a feminine and successful businesswoman.

It could be a person, a theme, a group of words, an archetype or even a country. Create your own filter to pass decisions through and have fun with it.

Day 8
Be chic in the summer

I have always found winter more of a chic challenge than summer, so much so that I wrote an entire book on how to survive the cold season. It's called 'How to be Chic in the Winter' and is still incredibly popular today; but I've had many ladies write to me and say, *When are you going to do 'How to be Chic in the Summer?'* and saying how they found it difficult to stay chic when the weather was so hot.

It can take me a while to write a book, so I thought I would include a chapter in *Thirty More Chic Days* and share what has worked for me in the meantime. I don't remember summers being so challenging, but maybe I've had my rose-tinted sunglasses on, showing summers as being balmy and effortless, because this past summer I did not find it easy at all! Perhaps part of it for me is my changing hormones 'at a certain age'.

I am in my late forties and I realized that I definitely felt different. Firstly, my weight seemed to be creeping up even though I was not eating that differently. Secondly, my core body temperature felt higher; in addition, I would have times during the day when I felt even warmer, like I'd been lit up from the inside. Thirdly, if I exerted myself too much (or even if I hadn't), I'd have palpitations quite easily. I felt somewhat relieved when I found out these were all symptoms of changing hormones.

Aside from all that though, I could see that past summers being looked upon with fondness *were* me viewing them through a tinted filter. Looking at the upcoming summer filled me with mild anxiety about how I could keep my healthy meals on track when daylight savings promoted the 'vacation drinks and nibbles' feeling every night. What was I going to do with my hair when it was humid outside? And most importantly, what was I going to *wear* on the hottest days, so I could still feel my chicest self?

Curate your summer wardrobe

The clothing aspect is the first one to focus on, because if we want to feel like we haven't given up on life, having at least a small selection of nice outfits to feel good in is a must. At the beginning of the season I look through my last year's summer clothes and see what I want to keep and what is looking a bit past it.

Depending on the item, I will repurpose clothes that are not looking their pristine best to home lounge wear. I'm not talking about clothes that have rips or stains, just that they no longer look quite so 'new'. If there is something that is damaged and cannot be mended or cleaned, I will either cut it up for cleaning rags or throw it out.

It's also 'interesting' to see how items fit from last year. I try not to freak out about it too much if everything seems a little snugger than I remember; it's a good reminder that sugar *is not* my friend, it just pretends to be.

The way I decide whether I am going to put an item away until next year or donate it now, is by asking myself whether I am excited to see that item. Can I imagine myself wearing it and feeling sexy and fashionable? Or is the highest praise I can muster up, 'Well it's still in good condition...' You will know that feeling when you get out your next season's clothes and think, 'Yay! I forgot about this; I love it!' Or perhaps it's more along the lines of, 'Urgh; I put this away last summer thinking it would magically become more appealing'. Spoiler alert: those pieces never do.

With these items it can be hard to let them go because it seems wasteful, but when I do make the decision to donate it feels like a weight has been lifted.

I am suddenly more excited about my closet when I don't have to make the decision to avoid wearing that ever-so-slightly frumpy top again. And the ridiculous thing about my procrastination is that someone else might be thrilled with that top and it will look amazing on them. Win/win!

Choose your favourite silhouettes

From previous summers I have decided that I am a dress girl rather than a skirt and top girl when it's too hot to wear jeans (which are my staple for most of the year). I like dresses that are semi-tailored and knee-length or slightly above. Because I am short-waisted it is better for me to have no waistline on my dress.

Think back to outfits you have felt great in and look for more of those. Maybe it's three-quarter pants and a blouse in a soft fabric. Maybe it's floaty boho dresses. I think it's great that with the different seasons we can explore different sides of our own personal style.

Have a play around with the capsule wardrobe concept and design yourself a chic seasonal collection that you can mix and match (or just find half-a-dozen dresses you can rotate like I do!).

For me, I've found that well-made tee-shirt dresses can be worn with flip-flops or wedge heels. I bought three the same in black, red and navy/white stripes from Banana Republic four or five years ago and they've just about done their dash now. I got so much use from these dresses and I'm glad that I bought all three colours at once. The fabric is slightly thicker than normal tee-shirt material (double-faced jersey is the official term), so they were able to be worn to more places than a thin tee-shirt dress which really is only good for over your swimwear.

I've also enjoyed wearing soft denimy-chambray shift dresses the past few summers. They are easy to wash and give a quick press (if at all); I can still feel like 'me' in denim and they go with my shoes and accessories which suit my jeans look.

Plus, they're quite hard-wearing and not so easy to tear which is useful when our little rescue dogs get a bit over-excited. One of my favourite blush-pink tee-shirts had a tiny hole plucked in the front from an enthusiastic doggy claw which was very upsetting!

Fun tip: Look at movies or television programs set in the summer to see how the actresses dress. A costume designer's job is to put together a wardrobe to reflect a character's personality, so if you like one outfit they are wearing, it's likely you will gain some new ideas from other outfits in the same movie.

Think 'cooling beauty'

I have wavy hair that frizzes in humid weather, and what I have found is good for hot, sticky days is to wash my hair and slick it back into a low bun like a ballet dancer would. To look polished, I like to roll a cotton scarf into a long ribbon and wind that around my bun a few times, finishing with a tiny knot.

Not only do I look (and feel) pulled together, but my hair being damp starts my day off on a cool note. I use a leave-in conditioning treatment, mousse or gel, so when I brush my hair out that night it feels silky and healthy.

If we have a day when it is not so humid and I'm at home, I like to let my hair dry naturally in waves. Later on, I might blow-dry around my hairline with a brush to finish off the look.

I also like to play around with other hairstyles that keep my hair off my neck such as stylish ponytails or experimenting with French braids (practice makes perfect!)

With makeup, I have found Estée Lauder's Double Wear foundation excellent on hot days. I let my SPF moisturizer soak in while I have breakfast, then blot with a tissue to remove perspiration from my skin (it's usually on my nose and upper lip when the weather is warm!). I then apply it with a sponge.

I have changed from using my fingers or a foundation brush to a Beauty Blender sponge and love it. I started out with a proper Beauty Blender and after a while when it no longer cleaned up as well, I tried a $4 cheapie which just as good. I'm glad I tried both price options otherwise I'd always have wondered. Sometimes cheaper versions of an item work fine, and sometimes they don't.

When it comes to body-care, I moisturize all over every day as I do in the winter, but in summer I add a gradual tanner to my beauty regime. I also wear SPF 15 moisturizer on my décolletage, because I can go quite pink there. I bought myself an inexpensive epilator which I use on my legs to free me from shaving them. Every so often I will shave my legs in between epilations because I find this helps exfoliate my skin and prevent ingrown hairs.

Eating well in the heat

The one saving grace of summer is that salads are more appealing than in the winter, when I crave stodgy, warm, comforting food. My top tip for eating healthy in the summer is to *prepare ingredients ahead of time*.

Having a vegetable chiller full of bell peppers, carrots, lettuce and other salad ingredients is great, but then you still have to wash and slice them. What I do now is have a chop-a-thon a few times a week where I fill GladWare or Tupperware containers with all manner of jewel-toned goodness. You could mix salad ingredients together so that you have one big container to ladle a portion into a bowl at lunchtime, or be like me and have smaller individual containers of ingredients. Doing it this way appeals; it feels like I am at a gourmet salad bar putting my lunch together.

I don't buy salads often, but when I do they always help me like salads more as well as give me new combinations to try. When I worked next-door to a Subway, I was inspired to recreate my own version of their salad at home. I'd have fresh vegetable ingredients ready to go, adding a topping of shredded cheese to my chopped cold roast chicken. I also invested in a lidded salad container to eat from, so I could pour my salad dressing on at the end and give the whole thing a good shake to mix everything together.

Plus, having a couple of lidded salad containers meant I could pre-make a few salads and then add the dressing right before I ate. The less barriers to eating healthy, the better.

But what about after work, when you get the vacation feeling as you arrive home in the blazing sunshine? I say take the vacation feeling all the way and pretend you aren't at home having to go to work the next day. Go for a stroll around the neighbourhood before dinner, read a book for a little while, then cook a tiny and exquisite steak on the barbeque to serve with green beans and new potatoes.

If you do have to do a load of laundry, do it after dinner while you are organising your clothes for the next day. I don't always set out my outfits the night before, but when I do it's fun to add the extra accessories or wear something a bit better than I normally might. Having more fun with my clothing choices brings about a vacation feeling for me as well.

Transport yourself to the South of France (or wherever that dream place is for you)

When I think about my summer successes, it's because I've prepared ahead of time. I find outfits that are comfortable and attractive to wear and I replicate them. I imagine what a rich and glamorous lady might eat on her yacht and I make that for lunch or dinner. I slick my hair back and dust a light coating of bronzer on my cheekbones, temples and the tip of my nose like I'm heading to downtown St Tropez to stroll around, browse the shops and maybe grab a coffee in a café.

I am still the Paris girl of my dreams; the only difference is that she has caught the high-speed train down to the South of France for her summer vacation! I dress and act accordingly, even though I am still living my normal life in my everyday surroundings in Hawke's Bay, New Zealand. Why not? I say.

Thirty Chic Days inspirational ideas:

Come up with a theme for your summer. As I have shared, I love the thought of my inner Paris girl heading off to the South of France for her summer season. Maybe yours is the NYC girl going to the Hamptons or your inner Londoner jetting to Spain.

Whatever the inspiration is for you, **let your inner stylista and happy girl guide you** through a fun and glamorous summer. Eat the juicy fresh foods she nudges you to prepare, enjoy your curated closet and have fun trying out summer hairstyles.

At the beginning of the hot season, **decide that this is going to be your best summer yet**, and it will be!

Day 9
Have a closet like Coco

Imagine if you could wave a wand and magically transform your wardrobe into a Chanel showroom – wouldn't that be fabulous?

Even if you thought, 'Well, I don't know if Chanel is really my style, I'm more of a casual dresser', you'd soon change your mind once you felt the hand-sewn pieces with exquisitely fitted shoulders, and a cohesive colour palette which meant you could wear everything with everything else. It truly would be a dream closet.

Sure, this might only be a fantasy, but what if we took Coco Chanel as our wardrobe muse and gained inspiration from her attitude and sense of style?

Coco designed and wore clothing *one hundred years ago* which would easily look current today. If anyone was a fashion visionary, it was she. Coco didn't worry that what she wanted to wear wasn't the norm; in fact, it was *far* from the norm.

While ladies around her dressed in tight corsets, awkwardly confining skirts and heavy, elaborate hats, Coco was comfortable. She wore unstructured, elegant knit fabric garments made from jersey material, which was usually reserved for the manufacture of men's underwear. She excelled in creating an effortless style of dress. She wore trousers when women *never* wore trousers. She chopped her long hair into a chic and simple bob which was the opposite of the hardly-ever-washed pinned-up styles of the day.

Coco drew inspiration from men's tailoring as well as the iconic English country style of dress. Despite using many masculine clothing elements and having a washboard figure with a *jolie laide* face (from the French, meaning 'ugly pretty'), she was extremely feminine though.

Her clothing designs were trimmed with grosgrain ribbon. She wore ropes of pearls to soften the stark look of a black dress. Coco reclined in cream silk pyjamas. There were no fusty floral nightdresses in her armoire! She created an elegant simplicity in everything she did.

Be unique

For you and me, we can borrow from Coco's legacy by deciding for ourselves what *our* signature style expresses. We can choose what lights us up and wear that. Who cares what other people think as long as *we* love it? Do you really want to copy everyone else? When you look around, most people dress simply to cover their body. Where is the fun, the flair, the panache? For me, I'd rather be inspired to look my best by Coco, not the next person in the street or what the shops are offering this season.

I get it that if you're going to work, paying the bills, doing the housework and looking after the kids that the last thing on your mind might be curating your personal style. I can certainly slip into the hum-drum myself, but I find that when I do take more care with my appearance and lavish attention and love onto taking care of my clothes, it spills over (in a good way) into other areas of my life.

It's easier to eat healthy, I naturally move more, I'm more creative and an all-round happy human being.

What if the way to a scintillating existence is by taking care of the details and committing to high quality in everything you do? Surely you must recall at least one time where you felt like a million dollars in the clothes you were wearing, whether it was at a formal event or in an everyday outfit that just felt like 'you'.

I've always adored the idealistic French girl's wardrobe, so why not fully embrace that for myself? Ballet pumps, blue jeans, a fitted jacket and a pretty scoop-neck top finished with a scarf: *très bon*!

When you decide what you really love, whether it's country bohemian, French chic or minimalist classic, throw yourself fully into your happy place. Come up with your perfect style fusion by mixing different genres. Refuse to consider anything unless it aligns with 'your' style. This can be done on a budget or by spending a lot. It's not about money, it's about being the editor of your closet.

When you please yourself about what you love to wear, it doesn't matter what styles are showing in the stores (unless they catch your heart, of course). You get to choose what you will add to your wardrobe and what you will say *non* to.

It is far easier to buy everything you see than shop discerningly, am I right? The difficult part is to have an eye which edits strictly. Strict might sound too disciplinary to bring pleasure, but it's being strict about what you love and strict about what makes your heart swell with joy.

When you're firm about keeping out the flim flam and the mundane you need never declutter again, because you adore everything you've brought into your life and your closet from here on in. By practising discernment and training yourself to say 'no' to mediocre choices, you will have a closet filled with clothes you love, and which express your inner style perfectly.

How Coco is that?

Devise your own colour palette

Something else I love about the Chanel style is that there is a definite colour palette to her look. When I think of Chanel I think of a black dress with a white camellia brooch and pearls. A navy suit with beigey-gold rope trim. Gilt costume jewellery. Tones of beige, cream and white worn together. Blush pink worn with red lipstick. And Coco not only used her signature shades to design her clothing ranges but based her entire life around them.

I like my wardrobe colours a little softer than Coco, so if I was to have a colour palette it would be:

Denim (to me denim is a colour!)

Black

Blush-rose pink

Mid-grey

Bright pastels such as warm coral-tangerine, mint green and rosy-peony pink

Greyed-navy

When I look at favourite pieces in my closet; the pieces I put on as soon as they are back from the wash, it is in these shades. If a colour makes me feel happy just looking at it (such as peony, rosy and coral pinks), or sexy and powerful (like black), it belongs in my own personal palette. What are those colours for you?

Be a mover and a shaker

Coco is also an inspiration to stop looking around at what others are doing and *do it for yourself*. I highly doubt, if the Daily Mail website had been around when Coco was alive, that she would have read it each morning with her café crème. *Non*, Coco would have been starting her day with a quiet coffee and her thoughts, deciding if she was going to go horse riding, meet a friend in a café or head straight to her atelier to start another design.

Rather than read about someone else who has started a successful business, she would go out and start her *own* business, such as her first boutique on Paris's Rue Cambon. She was a person who made things happen. She was a truly visionary lady who has impacted fashion and even the way we live, a century later. To be as gutsy as she was would be impressive now, but back then? It was outstanding.

Live your 'brand'

To me personal style is more than what you wear – it's about how you live your life.

I love the concept of creating my own 'brand' where everything is cohesive. It wouldn't feel good to me to wear beautifully tailored clothes when out, but slouch around at home on the sofa eating popcorn. Those two things do not go together!

By choosing how you want to live your life – starting with your closet – you can elevate every part of your existence to a frequency that makes you feel happy and successful every day.

Some may think it shallow to create your life on a foundation of chic personal style, but to me it makes perfect sense. It is enjoyable for those around you, but it's really for yourself. It makes *you* feel good. It inspires *you* to be your best, and it encourages *you* to be your most fulfilled self. This in turn inspires other people in your life and it's a beautiful upwards spiral.

In France it is accepted that you will dress and groom yourself well, not only for you, but because it is pleasant for others to see when you are in a public place. Isn't that a fabulous mindset? That everyone will add to the beauty of a place by making the most of themselves? It's your public duty!

Choose your flavour

Decide what inspires you and dive right in. Surround yourself with colours, textures, sounds and images that make you happy to be alive. Don't be like everyone else, be *you* unapologetically. With a twist of Coco for inspiration.

You don't need to tell anyone what you're doing either. Just for fun, keep your inspiration propagating in your secret garden and hug it to yourself as if it were propelling you along from within, because it is. I have found, to my detriment, that when I release my inner motivation to the world it can be dissipated and no longer has the same power for me.

Far better to interact with the world in a friendly and respectful manner and keep your inner style as your own driving engine. Can you imagine Coco announcing to her peers, 'I am going to be quite mysterious and unique with my clothing choices'. I can't either! Instead, she simply got on with her life, focusing on her next project and living in a way that suited her.

To complete this chapter, may I share with you my own personal Chanel-inspired philosophy? I wrote this as Chanel, then borrowed it for myself to keep the focus on how I wanted to evolve and it inspires me daily.

~~

I am full of ***confidence for my own creativity.***

I know that I can ***create a good living for myself*** *with my creativity if only I would believe in myself and stay the course.*

I am ***not swayed by others opinions*** *of what I can or cannot do.*

I remain ***focused on the kind of lifestyle I want to create for myself.***

I ***dare to dream****, and dream about big ideas.*

*I **do not waste time on unimportant things** that do not need my attention.*

*I do necessary jobs that don't thrill me in the **quickest possible time, and I do them well.***

*I **remain positive** about what I am adding to the world.*

*Food is delicious and nourishing, and mealtimes are social, but food is far down the importance scale for me. **I eat well, then I forget about food** until the next meal.*

*I **focus on one thing at a time**, I do not multi-task.*

*I work at something until I have finished it. I do not let my mind wander if a part becomes difficult. I work around it; tackle it from a different angle. **I persevere until I am done**.*

***Quality comes above all**. If something is worth doing, it is worth making a good job of without being a procrastinating perfectionist. If it is not worth quality work, then I question why I am doing it.*

*I am never afraid to put my work out there. **I take courage and show it to the world**.*

~~

As you can see, having Chanel as a closet muse goes far beyond clothes, at the same time as being all about what you wear. Borrow her confidence that what you want to wear is *exactly* the right thing for you. Be happy to own your unique style and employ decorative touches that suit *you*.

If Coco could do it a century ago, we can certainly do it today.

Thirty Chic Days inspirational ideas:

Use nostalgia as a guiding light. What did you love to wear as a child? As a teenager? Do any of those colours, pieces or styles appeal to you now? Many of Coco's iconic looks, such as the little black dress, were reportedly inspired by her life growing up.

From my childhood I loved to be feminine yet modern as well as casually elegant, and I prefer the same colours and scents as I did back then too – soft, pretty shades and floral fragrances.

Harking back to my younger years helps me hone in on what I love now, both by showing me examples of what I used to enjoy, as well as giving me permission to coddle my inner child; I find this comforting. I let her show me what I might want to include in my closet now.

Put together your own bespoke colour palette. What are your favourite neutrals and accents? What colours always appeal to you? Look in your closet and note down the colours of your favourite clothes. Include sleepwear and underwear in this – what shades jump out and make your heart sing? Write them all down or gather images online and from magazines to see how beautifully they all come together. Vow to bring more of these colours into your life.

On the flip side, find out what colours disappoint and weed them out. For me two come to mind – I love the idea of a crisp white shirt, but when I wear it, the starkness makes my hair and face appear orangey-yellow. I am far better in softer light-neutral shades such as oatmeal, beige and buttermilk.

I have also been caught out by dark charcoal grey because I love medium grey, but when I wear this colour it flattens not only my looks but my spirit too. It's close to black, greyed-navy and mid-grey which are all shades I wear well, but charcoal isn't good for me for some reason. Keeping this in mind (mostly) helps me bypass these shades when choosing something new.

Use your signature colour palette not only in your wardrobe, but for other areas as well: home décor, candles, writing paper – why not surround yourself with your favourite colours in every aspect of your life?

Day 10
From Paris to the South of France

I have had a love affair with France for a long time. When I was eleven- or twelve-years-old I studied the typical week of a French family. I have no idea why I chose this topic but there must have always been some fascination inside of me for the French lifestyle.

Fast forward to the present day, and I've been back and forth on letting my inner French girl run the show. I turned away from her for quite a while because I felt shamed by those who said, 'don't idolise the French, they're not perfect' and I did feel like I was following the crowd by glorifying the Paris lifestyle. One reviewer of my book *Thirty Chic Days* even called me delusional for this!

Then, one day I had the thought, *I don't care what anyone else thinks*. I don't care if I don't want to move to Paris or even learn the language. If bringing my own piece of *Francais* to my life here in New Zealand makes me happy, there's no harm in that.

The beauty of Paris and the charm of the idealistic French lifestyle has woven its magic over many throughout the years, so I know I'm not alone here. Perhaps you feel this too?

I have travelled to Paris once, and will go again. It is a city deserving of its devotees and I am so glad to have memories in my head of the steep Montmartre streets and elegant boulevards. But even if I hadn't, I could still concoct a potent cocktail to sip from as I spin her magic into my everyday life.

Paris brings out the best in me. She encourages me to effortlessly elevate my standards and choose from the perspective of my higher self. She helps keep frumpiness from my closet and faux foods from my pantry. My Parisian self sips a glass of wine or hot coffee instead of a diet cola. She takes the time to apply a light ten-minute makeup every day even if she has no plans to go anywhere.

Paris helped me recently to think differently about my shift in location. My husband and I had sold our home and business in the big city and moved with our two cats to the small provincial area where I'd grown up, a five- or six-hour drive from where we'd been living.

I love living where we do now and adore the slower pace of life. The orchards and vineyards that surround us are a nice change from motorways and intensive housing.

I was struggling with a few things though; my new identity as a work-from-home writer as well as getting into a productive and enjoyable routine. I was also evaluating my wardrobe style; I wanted to be comfortable and relaxed, but still feel chic and presentable because I see neighbours and family members most days.

French inspiration

My lightbulb moment came when I imagined myself as the chic Parisian lady of my dreams. It was as if she had moved from Paris to the South of France. And from that I had found my inspirational motif to assist in the smoothing over of my lifestyle adjustment.

This is helping me to curate my wardrobe season by season, as I add (and subtract) pieces of clothing that portray my ideal 'Paris femme in the South of France' image; mixing chic and elegant with a more casual way of life. I am still me and feel authentic, but I can tell you, it's fun to have this lens to focus through.

If anything, I have gone back to my young adult days where I enjoyed building my wardrobe with the classics – a crisp blouse, smooth ponytail, pearl stud earrings and a comfortable and well-fitting pair of jeans paired with ballet flats.

And because I spent seventeen years living in the city, I bring that to my new lifestyle too. The sophistication, appreciation for the arts and cinema, and being inspired to invite friends around for high-spirited dinners.

Imagining I am that chic Parisian who has now relocated to the warm and sunny climes of Saint Tropez or Provence all adds to the fun as I go about my usual day, and encourages me to dress a little better, maybe paint my nails and also decorate our home on a budget (décor mix: Ralph Lauren with a dash of French chateau).

I play French music softly in the background as I write my books and tend to my home. Lunches are often scrambled eggs with garden-grown parsley and my daily diet is full of fresh produce.

Be happy to be different to others

Yes, the French influence provides a lot of inspiration for me to enjoy a simple and beautiful life. It doesn't even cost me any more than if I had simply trudged along in a perfunctory manner.

Some of us are more inspired by beauty than others, and if those who don't mind a practical life want to call me delusional, I'd completely agree with their statement.

The meaning of the word delusional is 'a mistaken belief that is held with strong conviction even when presented with superior evidence to the contrary' and 'holding idiosyncratic beliefs or impressions that are contradicted by reality or rational argument'.

I think these descriptions are fabulous, and here's why. For some quirk of personality, I love being different to other people. I enjoy marching to the beat of my own drum and I adore setting my own ways of being.

It can be easily proven that I don't live in France and likely have no French blood in my veins. However, I enjoy creating elaborate fantasies for myself to pepper my everyday with fun. In my mind I live in a big snow-filled globe with magical glittery flakes surrounding me and infusing my life with joy and happiness.

I have no desire to live a boring, mundane life without any magic whatsoever. I'm guessing that if you enjoy my blog and books, you are the same. Isn't it fun to be this way? It's like we have a secret hug inside ourselves that enables us to do our work, deal with traffic and cook dinner all with a contented smile on our face.

We are carrying Paris around in our mind, and Paris carries us in return. And now, I have Provence and the South of France as inspiration too.

But how do I bring the essence of Paris and Provence to my life here in New Zealand? For me, it's all those little things that compound to bring about a bright and positive feeling of happiness, and this in turn elevates my frequency and makes my days seem more magical. Delusions of grandeur? Please bring them on!

Here are my favourite ways to do this:

- Playing French accordion tunes on my iPod, Paris café music from YouTube, Edith Piaf and soundtracks such as from the *Amélie* movie at home.

- Planting my favourite red-orange geraniums in terracotta pots outside. I co-planted a recent purchase with white tumbling lobelia, and a few rogue flowers were blue – so appropriate: the *Tricolour* national flag of France is blue, white and red.

- Upgrading my lingerie as needed, and purchasing lacy undergarments in pretty colours – they don't need to be expensive. My current bras are from K-Mart, and I ordered knickers from Victoria's Secret when they had a special offer, which they often do.

- Making meals that feel Francais to me: a bubbling casserole in the Le Crueset, tomato salad, rich chocolate mousse in tiny cups.

- Serving picky, nibbly meals outside on a big wooden board when it's warm: cheese and crackers, salami and cold roast chicken, capsicum slices, and sparkling water or wine in a carafe; what I imagine might be served in an out-of-the-way local café.

- Dressing with care each day, no matter what I'm doing, as well as being up-to-date with my grooming – legs are epilated or shaved, limbs moisturized every day, hair clean and styled. It really takes no extra money to do this, just effort and a little investment of time. I'd estimate it takes me no longer than fifteen minutes a day to do something small towards my grooming, and the compounding benefits mean that you will look – and feel – good with the minimum of effort if you do so regularly.

- Reading a classic book outside, with big glamorous sunglasses on. I could be in a public park, at a café or even at home – add a coffee and in my mind, I am sitting at a bistro table in Paris.

- People watching; looking for style inspiration; being out amongst everybody going about their day. Walking, seeing. Parking my car and walking a series of close errands achieves this, and I get some exercise in too.

- Being happy with my age and looking to European women who seem to be more relaxed about growing older than some of us. I love the concept of making the most of yourself with healthy foods and purposeful movement, positive thoughts, youthful and stylish clothing and fresh, minimal makeup where your skin tone shines through.

- Decorating my *maison* with touches of luxury such as gilt mirrors (bought inexpensively from charity stores and furniture auctions), candles, and cushions made from inexpensive offcuts of good quality fabric.

- Carrying an air of sexiness and insouciance around with me. It's not that I dress ultra-sexy, but by having an internal landscape of sexiness going on, it informs how I hold myself and what I choose to purchase. Sexy to me is fresh fruits and vegetables, champagne, clothes that feel good against my skin and help me feel confident, and drinking plenty of water all day long. Doesn't having an inner sexiness sound very French to you? It does to me.

- Taking inspiration from those pink and gold beauty boutiques in Paris (such as Annick Goutal), I stage my own cosmetic displays. A curated selection of everyday makeup in a pretty dish, having one or two perfumes displayed on a small silver tray alongside a rose in a bud vase, a pretty handcream by the bed... the ideas are endless.

- Going out with my husband on a date where we visit a hot new bar or have coffee together. Sure, most of the time we'll have a drink at home instead, but I find it so enjoyable to dress up and go out somewhere, even if only for an hour or two.

That's what I'm all about: enjoying where I live *and* adding a bewitching dusting of fairy-tale on top, like icing sugar over strawberries. Life is what we make of it, and I think we owe it to ourselves to enjoy every day as much as we can. Why on earth wouldn't we?

Don't get me wrong, I adore living in beautiful and sunny Hawke's Bay, New Zealand (I'm on the east coast of the north island) and doubt I will live anywhere else, but Paris is my spiritual home. French music transports me, I swoon when I come across someone with a French accent, and the French woman's style is truly covetable.

That's why I enjoy bringing in my own little French-style accents to make life fun.

Thirty Chic Days inspirational ideas:

Choose your inspiration. If Paris isn't your first true love, what is? Perhaps you are more an Italian Chic kind of girl, or Tokyo is your happy place. If you were offered a first-class ticket to anywhere in the world and could go tomorrow, where would you choose? Take *that* place and dream up an imaginary world for yourself.

Move there in your mind. How would you dress if you were visiting or even lived there? What kinds of activities would you do? How would you dine and what would you eat? Brainstorm a delicious list as long as you can make it and choose the most compelling point to enjoy today.

If where you live right now is your dream place, lucky you! What is it that you love about where you live and what do tourists rave about? Commit to bringing more of those thoughts and activity into your every day and remind yourself how lucky you are to live there.

And if someone calls you delusional? I say take it as a compliment.

Day 11
Honour your feminine heart

If you find that you are do-do-doing and go-go-going all day, it can seem like there isn't enough time for the pretty and dainty things in life. I often feel like that too, and I put off 'frivolous play-time' in favour of completing all the tasks on my daily list.

In doing this though, I find that I procrastinate doing my chores because I am not doing something more fun. Which in turn means my jobs can take me all day and then there really is no time for the more uplifting activities on my wish list. It's a bad circular loop that's for sure!

I changed this unhelpful habit pattern by indulging my femininity daily. It was all very well to want to enjoy my day more, but how could I go about it? It wasn't simply a matter of putting on lipstick or perfume; I needed to ask myself what would honour my feminine heart. What kinds of activities and small additions to my day would help me feel good and therefore be happier and more fulfilled?

When I did do something like have a professional manicure or massage, it felt hollow. Of course, it was nice at the time, but there wasn't a lasting effect. I'd spent money, I felt bad for the person doing it (truly!) and there were the hours out of my day with travel, parking, the treatment and getting home again.

I also often found that the appointments weren't as long as advertised. For example, my 'thirty-minute back-rub (allow forty-five minutes in total)' was abruptly wound up at twenty-two minutes, and my 'deluxe one-hour pedicure' was completed within three-quarters of an hour, with my foot and leg massage short and rushed.

Something that was meant to be an indulgent treat ended up being more of a stressor than if I hadn't had it done. And I'd paid money and spent time on it too!

Create your own feminine ways of being

I decided to brainstorm all the ways I could feel cosseted and relaxed without relying on other people or buying something. I asked myself what made me feel serene and ladylike and vowed to do as many of those things as often as I could.

I found that even just reading through my list had the effect of feeling soothed and tranquil. This in turn assisted me in being the softly elegant woman I desired to be.

I identified that I feel feminine when:

I have soft colours and textures around me
I eat water-rich foods
I am fragrant
My legs are smooth
My skin is soft
I move with grace
I stand tall and elegant
I rest often
I make food for my darling
I get 8-9 hours' sleep
I journal
I have boudoir time
I read Victoria magazine
My nails are filed and buffed
I wear handcream
I seduce my man
I eat fruit
I make soup
I am at home
I spend time with my lady-friends
I move my body
Our home is tidy, clean, neat and orderly
I play my relaxing music softly
I have an at-home facial
I eat healthily

I calm myself with pleasant thoughts
I breathe deeply
I am creative
I wear coordinating, pretty underwear
I treat my husband like a king
I am the queen of my life
I do stretches
I blow-dry my hair and wear makeup
I drink sparkling water or herbal tea
I spend time with my style files and inspiration documents
I speak my mind
I am gentle with myself
I move slowly and with poise
I enjoy pleasures such as reading
I spend time with my sewing supplies
I give myself time and permission to do what I love
I get up early so that I can enjoy hot tea with my current book before starting my day
I build in a buffer of time so I am never late for an appointment

I have brainstormed 'I feel feminine when...' many times, and while there are entries that come up over and over, there are also new ones.

Whether I am creating my list or choosing an item to inspire myself with, it feels like I am honouring my highest self – almost like I am following my own delicate and ladylike spiritual path. It feels so good, and this positive feeling helps me be at my calm and centred best.

When I am *not* in this frame of mind, I can easily go the other way entirely, heading for the base factor feel-good by watching reality television and eating snack foods. It might be fun to look forward to and it certainly starts out as enjoyable, but these activities quickly descend into regret and remorse. They are definitely faux pleasures when done as escapism.

Sure, there are many times when I have watched a reality television programme and felt inspired by it rather than like an unmotivated loser – I'm sure you can recognize those times for yourself too: one activity leading to two opposite feelings.

When I ask myself what would feel good, as with my inspiration list above, it's like I am following my natural path and living the way I am meant to live. If simply perusing my list feels good, then doing those things will be even better. I feel light as a feather and more feminine and attractive (not only to others, but to myself).

By nurturing yourself this way you will not so readily turn to other forms of nurturing that can be harmful when done with the wrong intention or to excess, such as shopping or eating.

I use these ideas for those times when life seems out of kilter – when I spend more time online than is good for me or when I multi-task and rush (which never produces good results or calm feelings). I can feel comforted by my idealistic desired ways of being which are always there for me.

Intentionally choosing your feminine life

Coming back to these things recognizes and shapes my wish for a simple and peaceful home life. I enjoy structuring my days so that I have time for my relationship with my husband, tending to and enjoying my home, writing and other creative work such as sewing and knitting.

Of course, I still do other jobs such as laundry, tidying and cleaning, grocery shopping and cooking, and banking/finances, but when I make time for enjoyable pastimes I don't mind doing the chores as much. It's almost as if my feminine pursuits help me feel lighter and everything else flows from that.

Instead of getting up in the morning and launching straight into my dirty washing or weeding the garden, I start with a hot cup of tea in bed with a book, and my journal beside me. During the half-hour it takes me to finish my tea, not only have I read a chapter or two, but I have journaled some inspiration for the day. Having that half hour feels luxurious, and it takes from nothing from my day, because I decided to rise a half hour earlier to do so.

For those of you who are more night owls than morning people, take an extra half hour for your own quiet time before you go to bed. Maybe you will turn the lights out half an hour later, or you could decide to retire a half hour earlier to find that time.

Feminine chic mentors

Another way to inspire your feminine heart is to look at those women you admire, either in your real life or as public figures. What attributes do they have that you could bring the essence of into your own life?

Even though she has a much more polished Park Avenue personal style than I do, I am always inspired to be more feminine by Aerin Lauder. I don't desire to dress as she does or live as formally, but there are many details that I love to bring into my life thanks to her.

Think about someone who often inspires you and note down what it is about them that you feel uplifted by. Then, use this as a basis of what you can bring into your own life, in your own style, to create a similar feeling.

When I did this with Aerin, I came up with:

- Sleek and simple personal style
- Chic, polished and ladylike
- Family focused
- Unfussy
- Luxurious lifestyle
- A balanced life of family, work, play
- Hardworking and professional
- Good at what she does

- Takes her work seriously
- Down-to-earth
- Seems well-mannered and quiet
- Has followed her dream to create her own range
- Slim and healthy looking
- Feminine and elegant
- Rose pink and gold brand colours
- Floral fragrances
- Spa time, boudoir time
- Upper East Side
- Wealth, travel, luxury
- Décor style like a five-star boutique hotel

These descriptions and phrases encourage me to be my best self – elegant, focused and with a strong work ethic. I am inspired by women who have made their success in a feminine way.

And that's the great thing about creating your own inspiration by identifying what lights you up: you get to choose what is right for you. Follow what feels good and do more of it. When something feels icky inside, look at why and see how you can do things differently.

When you realize there is no perfect blueprint to the ideal life, it gives you such freedom to be yourself and create your own path. Customize *everything* to suit yourself. Browse around for ideas and see what is working for other people, then decide what belongs in *your* beautiful lifestyle.

Honour your own feminine heart and you can't go wrong.

Thirty Chic Days inspirational ideas:

Let there be time in your day for pleasurable activities. With any new habit I want to embed, I print off a single sheet with a month's worth of squares numbered 1-30 on it. I note my desired new habit at the top of the page and then aim to mark off each square daily. This month's habit is writing a new blog post within thirty minutes, and also writing my current book (this one!) for thirty minutes. When I have done both these things, I cross off the day's square.

It is amazing the effect accountability has on you. For me, it's worth completing the month not only to see my results and feel good about myself, but just as much to avoid having that calendar page mock me if it was left half empty!

Why not use the same technique to enjoy a feminine activity each day and see how good you feel after thirty days of doing so? You could choose one thing to do each day, such as thirty minutes reading a book for pure pleasure, or you could have a number of choices available, picking what you felt like on the day. (See my list at the beginning of this chapter, or you may have brainstormed your own.)

Your list to choose from might be:

Thirty minutes of reading
Enjoy one serving of fresh fruit
Have a home-facial with mask

Go for a half-hour stroll outside
Thirty minutes to do absolutely nothing

It would be fun to brainstorm a list of thirty and do something different each day too.

PS. No guilt is allowed. You are doing this for the good of *everyone* in your life because when you martyr yourself, no-one wins – I know this from frequent experience!

Day 12

Be easy to get along with

I'd like to share with you one of my secrets to happiness; something which has allowed me to be more content with myself, meet new friends easily, and attract my dream life to me in a seemingly effortless way.

I began to cultivate this attribute years ago and at first it was hard, but now I find it easier to uphold. Mind you, it's something I won't ever take for granted and will always be aware of. I want to become more of this over time, not less.

That quality? I desired to be someone who is an easy-going, pleasant and positive person who travels lightly through life and enjoys a happy-go-lucky disposition.

This was not my natural state back then; I thought that being cynical and sarcastic was amusing. I didn't want to be seen as a pushover so I had a barrier up. When I let that front down and started being nicer, life was better.

When I am like this, I am not a pushover and a people-pleaser as I feared I might become. Instead, I have found that being someone who is easy to deal with makes *life* easier. People prefer to connect with nice people. They'll remember you and possibly give you better service in the future. And even those who give you poor service can change if you show up as your best self. The great thing is, you'll hardly notice bad service when you are in this state of mind.

'Treat them mean, keep them keen' is not a good life motto, at least not for me. It feels so much better to be positive and cheerful, and nice and normal. There's no need to be a smarty-pants, people *just want nice*.

Find your potent combination

I didn't want to be bland and vanilla though, so I developed what I think is an unbeatable combination: combining being easy-going with what makes me uniquely me: dialling up the loveliness and adding to it a sparkliness that comes from my personality.

And it's something anyone can do. I was inspired to develop in this direction by coming across people who demonstrate this attribute. They are friendly and nice as well as being self-possessed. They own their inimitable ways of seeing the world and have you so caught up in their vortex that you just want to be around them.

Being more of who you are and sharing what truly makes you happy will do that. Not only will you find yourself being invited to more events, but you will also be content with your own company.

This is what I didn't realize when I was the 'sarcastic humour' type who saw every detail or flaw in a situation – it wasn't making me happy. I was constantly looking around for perfection and because life is not like that, experiences often fell short for me. This lessened not only my enjoyment, but my husband's too (because I'd always share my thoughts with him).

Think about people you admire in real life or celebrity-land (or even a book or movie character) who are kind, happy and easy-going. And then see what makes them stand out from others. I always enjoy watching Anne Hathaway in movies: she is upbeat and lovely as well as being slightly awkward and clumsy which I find endearing.

Of course, this is her acting, I don't know what she is like in real life, but who ever said you had to get your inspiration from real life? Someone dull, no doubt.

I would consider my potent combination to be this:

- Kind, sweet and caring

- Easy to live with

- Low-maintenance and down-to-earth

- Creative and sparkly
- Joyous, playful and child-like in my enthusiasm
- Positive and happy – I see the good in things
- Optimistic – expecting the best to happen and expecting the best from other people

I know this sounds like a pretty perfect person (well it does to me) and I'm certainly not like this all the time. I have my moments when I'm grumpy or short-tempered, but as much as possible I aim to be that positive, easy-going and enthusiastic person.

Not only have I been inspired by a few people in my life that it's easier to be successful that way, but it just *feels better*. It feels good to be happy! I get out of my own head, take action on projects and reach out to friends.

All in all, it's a good thing to be nice + be you.

Let people meet you at your level

Being who you are regardless of those around you is important as well. When you uphold your own high standards, it means that others will often meet you there.

The alternative is that you may be influenced by someone who is grumpy or sour, and dip to their level. This could leave both of you unhappy, whereas the first scenario leaves you happy, and the other person possibly uplifted by their interaction with you. Even if they stay the same, you are content and that's going to serve you well.

It's a key defining moment of life when you realize that you can choose your own emotional state; you don't need to be at the mercy of others' moods. For me, I choose to be pleasant, kind and upbeat, while still being strong on the inside.

Getting along with others is key to being successful in many areas of your life. Can you think of a work colleague, acquaintance, or friend-of-a-friend who you didn't particularly like because they were somewhat prickly? I certainly can, and I've probably been that person myself many times.

These days, as much as I can I aim to be accommodating, friendly and better with things such punctuality and getting back to people in a timely manner. I used to be so good with punctuality, but I've found myself slipping which doesn't feel good. When you are meeting with someone or they are coming around to visit and they are late, you don't feel as important.

It's the same getting back to someone if they've sent you an email or text message. My brother mocked me a few times for replying to his emails so quickly (insinuating in a joking way that I didn't have a life), so I started not responding to emails straight away. But then there's the risk of those messages becoming buried (which did happen), so I think I shall ignore my brother's ribbing and respond immediately if I want to.

Give bad news courteously

Even if you must give bad news or say no to somebody, you can do so in an agreeable way. When we had our retail business a customer might ask for a discount on a pair of shoes that were new on the shelves that day, for example. Instead of saying 'Are you kidding me?', I'd respond with, 'I wish I could help you out, but that shoe is new season stock. We have some sales shoes over here that are similar though, or these ones aren't as expensive.'

I'd be nice, and offer an alternative if I could. Even if I didn't have any other offer, just 'sorry no', there's no reason to be smart about it, and I'd always start with the 'I wish I could, but...'

That way the customer isn't embarrassed for asking. Have you ever had an experience where you've been made to feel silly in a restaurant or store? I have, and it doesn't leave you with good feelings about that establishment.

What about when you have to make a complaint about something though? I believe you can still be kind, positive and strong. It's not a case of being nasty or else a doormat. You can smile while getting your point across and the person you are talking with will likely go further than they might have than if you were horrid. I always like to include the phrase 'I really hope you can help me out with this' and it works well.

But what about something personal; say you've been invited to an outing that *just isn't you*. You don't have to tell them how you really feel about attending home sales parties, you can simply reply, 'Oh I'm sorry, I'm not available to come'.

It's gotten to a funny stage with my mum, because she loves live theatre and opera, whereas I... don't. She'll ask me (jokingly) if I want to go to a classical concert and I'll say, 'Sorry, I'm busy'. 'But you don't even know what night yet!'... 'I'm busy every night for that concert'. It always makes us both laugh; I mean, why not take your humour where you can get it!

My mum is someone who is easy to get along with. She is always in good spirits, doesn't have 'moods', is up for an impromptu coffee or lunch at any time and while she used to be chronically late, is now almost always on time. No, she's not perfect (sorry mum) but you can forgive a lot when someone has a friendly nature and goes with the flow.

Thirty Chic Days inspirational ideas:

Be the kind of friend you'd like to attract. This reminder encourages me to email or call friends to meet up instead of waiting for them to contact me. I remember birthdays and important dates such as a big medical check-up if they have mentioned it to me.

Make a decision that **you are a person who cruises through life**, enjoying yourself in a low-drama way.

Look at areas of your life where **you know you are high maintenance** and see if that is making you happy or if you want to change a few things.

Be punctual. As mentioned in this chapter this is something I am struggling with at the moment, and it's really bothering me because I used to pride myself on being punctual. Being on time shows a basic form of respect for the other person and I want to do that. It is far less stressful too.

We recently moved to live in a new area, and I think it's because I don't know the timings well enough for getting somewhere, but with the map app on my iPhone telling me how many minutes to my destination, I really have no excuse. I commit to you now that this is an area I will improve upon.

Day 13
Become a chic success

I adore the world of chic where I can dream of bringing my inner French Girl out to play. Then there is the other side of me: she is a go-getter, coach-yourself, personal development enthusiast who devours business building books and is always looking to better herself (in a fun and feminine way of course).

I *love* marrying up these two parts of myself and I can't help the personal development side coming out in my blog posts and books – it's as much a passion of mine as an elegant personal style and luxe yet laid-back living.

I get so excited when I read motivational books that rev me up and get me going. It's the best feeling in the world when a message hits you in the right place and you effortlessly take *off*.

It really is incredible when you receive a hit at the perfect time – the tipping point if you like – which ignites a spark into a flame. You're racing along, being amazing, achieving great things in small amounts of time. (I hope you find moments like this in my books too!)

It's a strange thing though: most people aren't willing to do what it takes to be successful. Sure, they might say they want to do something such as write a book, find a new job or declutter their home once and for all, but are they willing to put in the effort? Often not. Of course, I know *you* are not like that.

I had a friend-of-a-friend email me a while back to ask how I had written my books and built my online readership because she'd heard I was doing quite well (this was before I had created my training program on creating your dream life as a successful author). I wrote to her and shared all the steps I'd taken and asked what she planned to write about.

She replied and told me how busy she was and that she wanted to write a book but didn't have the time – she actually provided a long list of reasons why she was never likely to write her book. I was quite dumbfounded and wondered why she had sought me out for advice. Maybe she thought I had a magic answer that didn't involve her writing? Aren't people interesting!

For me, it's not about finding the time; it's finding the *motivation*. When I am inspired to do something it effortlessly comes ahead of other activities such as watching television or mindless Internet browsing. When I find myself lit up because of something I've read or listened to, or I've had a lightbulb-bright-idea-moment *I can't wait* to get cracking on a project.

Be a one-percenter

I know you are not that person who wishes and hopes she could be successful but can't really be bothered. You want to be different to others. You are not mediocre! You know that you want to break out of the hum-drum mould that most people are content to reside in.

And it's not like it takes that much effort either. If you decide you are going to dedicate an hour a day, or four hours a week (whatever suits your schedule) to a project, you will be further ahead in three months than most people would be in three years.

The simple truth is that most people would rather *consume* than *create*, and I can still find myself falling into that trap if I'd not mindful about it. Sometimes I realize it's been a few days or a week that I haven't written anything and it's hard to get started again; I've been consuming other people's information in the form of books – both fiction and non-fiction, podcasts, blogs and YouTube videos instead of creating my own inspiration and material.

On the other hand, when I start off my day by choosing to write for thirty to sixty minutes, it provides momentum. I find it easier to write and my mind pops out new ideas all the time.

Far from feeling deprived when I am up writing at 6 a.m. while most people are snoozing, or writing on a Saturday afternoon when others are out shopping and coffee-ing, I feel amazing. I am exercising my creativity and it feels incredible.

I love being different to 99% of the population, because when you look at how 99% of the population lives, they don't seem too inspired or happy with their lot. They are simply plodding through their days, self-medicating with food, drink, shopping and television until one day they'll die.

And then they complain that nothing exciting ever happens for them!

I know that sounds kind of rude and judgemental, but sometimes it's a tough love kind of thinking that is required to be successful. Please don't get me wrong, I certainly love food, drink, shopping and television too, but when I indulge too much at the expense of creativity and motivation it doesn't feel good at all.

The key is to enjoy everything in its place *and* be a person who creates their own luck and their own beautiful life.

Do you desire to live a mediocre existence or would you rather live in a way that makes you feel alive, excited, creative and abundant? Why not make a decision today that *you are a person who makes things happen?*

Don't look to the normal person when you are designing your life; look to the ones who are making successes of themselves and doing great things (and by great things, I don't just mean building skyscrapers; great things can be small things too). You will find inspiring examples everywhere – in your real life, online and by observing well-known people too.

Draw a line in the sand and claim that from this day forward ***you are a chic success***. It's a fun thing to think about: 'If I was a chic success, what would my life look like?' and note down everything that rings your bell. You'd then have a highly motivating customised blueprint as to how best to live your life.

If I asked myself that question I'd have thoughts such as:

- *I would be in premium physical health by eating for nutrition, stretching often, walking outside daily and doing short YouTube workouts at home.*

- *Where I live would be organized, tidy and welcoming, portraying a décor style which makes me fall in love with my home every day.*

- *I would release new book titles regularly and keep in touch with my audience, who feel more like friends. I would write towards my books every day for at least an hour.*

- *I would have peace of mind by trusting in the future and a higher power. I would eliminate worry, fear, shame and guilt.*

- *I would amplify my natural strengths and learn to work with my weaknesses (strengths: creative thinker, kind, easy-going – weaknesses: hard to focus sometimes, procrastinator, self-doubt).*

- *I would prioritize the important things in my life and take that down to a daily level, so I don't get caught up in busywork and doodle through my days not getting anything done.*

- *I would have fun curating all the details of my life such as my closet.*

- *I would take the time to journal regularly to make sure I am living in alignment with my true self.*

- *I would not be afraid to make changes – both big and small – so that I am always living in my most authentic way.*

Now, reading through this you might get the sense of 'It's all about her!' and you'd be right.

If I've learned one thing in all my years of reading personal development books, it's that you can only change yourself. Not your husband or your sister or your best friend. You might clearly see what they need to do but will they thank you for your unsolicited advice? Well, I think you already know the answer to that one!

How do I know this? It's a little embarrassing to say, but it's something I have done many, many times and I now have to almost tape my mouth closed and simply smile instead when I want to give someone my 'helpful' advice.

It's pretty rude when you think about it; who am I to tell another what to do? Am I so perfect that I think I can shower those around me with my pearls of wisdom? (The answer to that is 'no', by the way.)

It's not selfish to focus on self-study. By working on yourself and doing your best to live your most successful life, you are contributing to the world around you. By improving your own reality, you will not only be more available to those you love (because you are not struggling with your own limitations), but you will unintentionally inspire them to raise the standards of what they are willing to accept in their lives as well.

Have you ever met someone at a social event and been so knocked out by the energy and enthusiasm for life that seems to shine from them that it inspires you to make a few changes in your own life? I have, and it's a beautiful thing.

I believe these instances are sent to us so that we can elevate our own experience. I'm always on the look-out for them now, and, I aspire to have that sort of effect on others by living my best and most authentic life as well.

These lightning bolt moments can happen in both big and small ways.

A major example for my husband and I was having dinner with friends a few years back when one couple announced they'd rented out their house and were travelling for twelve months. One of their jobs was kept open, and the other left their job confident that they could get another one when they returned. This inspired us to sell our business and home to move from the city to a small country area six hours away because we'd always dreamed of doing it 'one day'. Now we are here and loving our new life.

A small example was when we had takeaway Thai food with our new neighbours recently. With all the plastic containers laid out, instead of using normal spoons to dish up, our neighbour brought out a collection of ornate and oversized vintage serving spoons instead. I wanted to emulate this for myself because I thought it was such an elegant and fun touch.

I visited our local auction house the following week and happened to see a box lot which included several large vintage serving spoons, and I got it for only $5! Isn't it funny how the Universe works? I would never have looked at that box lot if it wasn't for our shared Thai dinner and now I love our new vintage serving spoons (and you can call me Single White Female if you want to!).

When I dream how I want my 'chic and successful life' to be, it encompasses all parts of my existence – what kind of job I work in, how I live, what I wear, my habits and routines, who I associate with and how I spend my days.

It's a fun thing to think about all those different categories of your life and decide what your standards are for each. Most of us drift along like a boat without oars, being taken wherever the current is flowing. But what if we decided how we felt most successful and then steered ourselves towards that? How much more satisfying would that be?

The great bonus is, you can make it as ease-filled as you like. For me, I need fun, frivolity and lightness in my self-development, otherwise I look for it in other ways (like chocolate!).

When I figure out the easiest and most fun way to do things I still get done what needs to be done, but I fit in daily silliness with my husband and pets, read something enjoyable and generally enjoy my life.

I know when you have a long commute, family to clean up after and long hours at a job, being a chic success may be the furthest thing from your mind – you are just looking at getting through the day! – but what's the alternative? Slogging away until you look up and see that most of your life has passed?

Please promise me that you will take the time to allow yourself to add to your life in small ways to start with. And then, you might decide that you do desire this big change and you're going to look at how you can take the first steps towards that.

Perhaps it might be moving to a different location like I did, or wanting to work part-time instead of full-time. Maybe you want to get back into making your own clothes like you did as a teenager.

Brainstorm all the things that would make you feel happy and like a chic success and see what jumps out at you as the most exciting. What can you do towards that thing today?

Thirty Chic Days inspirational ideas:

Be a creator, not just a consumer. See where you can add value to your life by building things with your mind or your hands, your talents and your skills. You might think, 'I'm not a very creative person', but creativity covers a huge area. A great place to look is to see what is easy for you that others compliment you on.

Decide that you are not available for a mediocre life. What areas in your life have you been 'just putting up with'? Is there something easy you can elevate today? Often it's not about spending money either, it's about your intention and effort.

One area that comes to mind for me is my hair. I'm often just too lazy to spend the twenty minutes it takes to blow-dry it nicely every two or three days after I've washed it. I'll make the effort for special occasions, but surely my everyday life deserves the same care?

Often I'll not do things like this because I think it will take me too long and I don't have the time, but when I set a timer to see how long these dreaded tasks take, I'll always find it's much shorter than I think. With this information there is a smaller block to overcome the next time I am tempted to skimp on that task.

Claim being a chic success and make all decisions from that place. Lift your thoughts up from the melee of your everyday and brainstorm how you can live better and have more fun. Be your own conductor of the orchestral masterpiece that is your life.

Put the grand plans into place and let everything else fit in around them. Too often we put all the little things in first and then find no room left for what's important to us. It's similar to booking a vacation – you work around it because it's already there, whereas if you waited until the month you wanted to go away to book it, you'd find that you've got too much on to even think about going on holiday.

Strike while the iron is hot and make some changes... today!

Day 14
Grow better every year

When I turned forty several years ago I realized that I was entering the second half of my life. Certainly I plan to live longer then eighty (as much as one can plan for that kind of thing), and hope to be well into my nineties or beyond before I move on, but turning forty started me on this train of thought.

Suddenly, subjects such as menopause and retirement weren't abstract concepts for 'old people', but in my future. It was then that I decided I wanted to change what I thought this time of life was about. Rather than 'old', I was instead going to be a 'woman of a certain age'. I was going to become more youthful over time instead of the opposite. I was going to have fun and enjoy myself rather than wait patiently to fulfil my time here on earth.

A lot of people are negative about aging, and often they have so many good things happening in their lives but they just don't see them. I know that health can be an issue as you age, but I also think if you focus on 'this will happen when you get older', it will.

I've decided that my way of advancing through life is to *get better with age*. It's my guiding motto and one that I plan to fully embrace every day. *I am becoming better every year*, much like a fine wine or a lovingly tended vintage motor car!

I also plan to get richer with age, healthier, and slimmer. Of course there is much that is out of my control, but I believe people give too much weight to that side of things. There is a lot within our control, both physically and mentally. And mentally is where it's at: when you think youthful thoughts, are positive and focus on the good, I believe you can feel younger.

And when you treat your physical self well, you can feel more youthful too. I know myself when I eat badly that I am more likely to have headaches. When I skip my daily walks I feel less motivated. When I spend too long sitting on the sofa I feel stiff. Aches and pains can bother me if I go to bed late, eat too much sugar and dwell on negative thoughts.

But when I walk daily for at least half an hour, do some stretches on the floor, drink lots of water, eat good protein and plenty of fresh fruits and vegetables, go to bed at a reasonable hour and focus on good posture, I feel *so well*.

These are simple and free improvements to my life that I can add in one at a time and have them become habits. Whenever I have a habit that I don't like and would like to change, I think to myself: 'How is my life going to be in five years' time if I keep this same habit?' It makes it easier for me to do something different and not feel too deprived when I reframe it like that.

Be inspired by others who are older than you

I see what my future could be like by observing those around me. I see that I could continue with the comfortable habits I have, and grow into a matronly, frumpy figure with increasing health issues.

Alternatively, I also see examples of women who have taken their health into their own hands and become or remained trim and vibrant well into retirement.

I see men and women who mill around doing not much at all, like they have all the time in the world, and others who have new adventures, both big and small, every year. There are two quite extreme examples of the adventurous type in my own family.

My father, at 73, is currently in the United States where he is planning to compete for his second record at the Bonneville Salt Flats speed week in September. That's right, his second speed record. He set the first one last year when he raced his vintage Triumph motorcycle on the salt.

And my great aunt, now in her eighties, joined a group expedition through Nepal attempting to reach the Mt Everest base camp a couple of years ago. Apparently, she was quite a hit with the Sherpas who had never had anyone so old on their trip – they proudly told her that!

These two are so inspiring to me as to what you can achieve no matter your age, and they encourage me to ignore others' opinions and do whatever *I* want to do. 'Have big dreams' is what I'd take from their example.

Neither of them are particularly wealthy, but I've observed that they have prioritized spending so that they can indulge in what is important to them. Both live a frugal and simple home life, and save money for their trips.

My great aunt in particular has travelled her whole life and spent the minimum amount of money on her lifestyle so that she could continue her passion for travel. Every trip she goes on she says 'that's my last trip'... and then books another. She just can't help herself! Currently she is on a group tour in the Northern Territory of Australia.

As far as their health goes, they ignore what they can and deal with the rest. It is rare that I will hear either of them talk about any health issues that they might have.

We don't have to climb a mountain or race a motorcycle at 100 miles per hour though. I probably won't do either of those things either. But there are many other ways we can embrace our life as we age, rather than complain about how old we are getting and regale others with our aches and pains.

There are projects, hobbies, gardens, books, marathons; so many fun things to give our lives structure, purpose, meaning and satisfaction.

I have certainly been guilty of wasting the precious time I've been gifted on this earth, so please know that I am writing this chapter as much for myself as for you. I had a blast in the first half of my life and my goal is to make the second half *even better*.

Reinvent yourself by embracing change

I used to be someone who was proud of their old mobile phone (which only made calls and sent text messages). I loved paper books and shunned anything digital. Kindle schmindle. I was proud of my old-fashioned-ness.

What changed? I was given an example of how aging being like this could be. I am happy to be inspired by tradition, but I came to see that I felt quite stuck at my blanket ban on anything 21st century. But why couldn't I do both? Why was I sticking doggedly to my black or white decision?

The example that shook my world was an elderly well-dressed gentleman who came shopping in our store a few years back. He was purchasing shoes for his grandson and wanted to check the size required. Pulling a smartphone out of his jacket pocket, he tapped away. He messaged his grandson and had an answer within seconds.

At the cash register, he realized he had to transfer some money to pay for them. 'Would you like to use our telephone?', I asked him. 'I'm good thanks', he replied, as he whipped out his smartphone again and shifted funds around instantly. 'All done', he said with a smile.

This one incident opened my eyes and made me declare to myself on the spot, *I want to be like you when I grow up*. His whole persona vibrated with a youthful energy. He was clearly the age he was, but he was also vibrant and quick moving, both brain-wise and physically.

This gentleman helped me change my mind in an instant, and I decided to One. Upgrade to an iPhone, and Two. Become someone who learned about new technology instead of shunning it or feeling fearful of advancing changes in how things are done.

In addition, I have found that keeping up with new technology not only helps you feel more youthful, but it's good for your brain. Much like puzzles, learning new things activates your grey matter and keeps all the cogs ticking over in your head nicely.

I imagine someone who is steadfastly stuck in the past like I used to be, having their mind harden like concrete, whereas someone who is interested in learning new things will have an elastic and supple mind. There is truth to that, because 'plasticity' is quite the buzzword these days to do with using our brain well.

I've also expanded this to staying loosely in touch with younger pop culture: movies, books and music etc. This helps keep me feeling young too. I'm not trying to be one of the kids but it is invigorating to know what they are talking about.

As for an e-Reader, I am currently engrossed in a paper book, *and* I love having my Kindle in my bag at all times in case I have to wait somewhere. It's so aging when you hear someone say, 'Oh. I couldn't read from a Kindle, I love reading from *paper*', but I used to say *the exact same thing all the time*.

It feels so strange that I was staunchly anti-tech, until one day I wasn't. But that's the thing about being youthful of spirit too – you are always free to change your mind. Change is freeing, change is youthful, change will revitalize you.

Thirty Chic Days inspirational ideas:

Decide that your life is only going to **get better every year** from now on. I've had people say that I'm only lying to myself and that I have to face up to reality. But I didn't say I'm going to get *younger* every year. I'm going to get *better*.

Aging is inevitable (and far preferable to the alternative), but do we have to think about it all the time and simply wait for it to happen? Instead, let's get busy loving and living our fabulous life.

Here are my far more appealing options than moaning about getting older, talking about poor health and how things are only going to get worse:

- Deal with any health issues you can, and ignore the rest as much as possible. Don't talk about them; this only amplifies them.

- Be in as good a health as you can. Look to your future self and see how vibrant and joyous she is because she has cultivated health-supporting habits over the years. Far from feeling deprived, she's having the time of her life.

- Declutter so as not to stay stuck in the past. You don't want to feel weighed down by your possessions. Your desired outcome is to feel joyously light and unencumbered.

- Don't joke about everything going downhill, both for your own state of mind as well as how you come across to others. Every word we speak affects us. I've had reading glasses for a couple of years now, and it's no big deal. However, I have also seen many examples of people rummaging around in their pockets and making a big deal out of finding their glasses as they declare 'I can't see a thing without these now, just another sign I'm getting older'. I don't see the need to say that at all; get your glasses out and start reading the menu, no fuss necessary! Not only will you look a lot more cool, calm and collected but you're not filling your mind with rubbishy thoughts that will certainly ensure you age far quicker.

- Go lightly with your clothing purchases each year so that you don't have a huge investment you won't want to let go of. Buy what you need for that season, if you need anything at all. Wear and enjoy it and move on when that item is looking less than pristine. Use this as a chance to update your wardrobe each season with a few items that you require, and which will also help you feel fresh and modern.

- Own your choices – for example: not colouring your hair or colouring hair. I didn't have artificial colour in my hair for many years and was happy with that, then one day I felt drab. I've been having blonde highlights ever since and feel great about it.

  Another example is that I didn't drink alcohol for over five years after reading a library book that flicked a switch I didn't know needed flicking. Then, one day I woke up and decided I wanted to drink wine again (and I started that night). Whatever choices you make, own them.

- Look as good as you can *for you*. Enjoy your wardrobe. Wear makeup if you want to. I'm enjoying makeup more than I ever have now, and I enjoy putting on a little bit each day. It feels like an artistic expression and makes me happy, even if I'm not leaving the house.

- If you've always wanted to try Botox, why not? I haven't, but I did have minor eyelid surgery a few years ago and I *love* the results. I've always been happy with everything else about me, but I'm so happy that I took that leap.

- Change how you are in the world – why not reinvent yourself? Create an ideal picture and see how you can move towards it. Not in an 'I'm not good enough' sense but more a 'Let's see how amazing we can make life' kind of way. I do love a good makeover, and how much fun does it sound to reinvent yourself? I think there are many ladies who are looking to do this. Maybe they have more time now their children are grown.

I've had to change a lot myself as I've transitioned from city-life and full-time work in our business, to living in the provinces and working from home as a writer. At first I struggled, even though it was what I'd been working towards for many years. I had to formulate a daily schedule for myself, recreate my wardrobe so I could feel comfortable and presentable every day, and upgrade my thoughts on what it meant to work from home.

Change isn't comfortable, but it can be the making of us and bring a lot of joy if we let it. And, it keeps us young!

Day 15
Elevate your dining experience

I love to find tweaks in my life that are easy and simple yet make a big difference to my daily life and how I feel.

Something I started several years ago which has helped elevate my dining experience, was to use cloth dinner napkins at all mealtimes. Even if were eating pizza in front of the television, we had cloth napkins on our laps.

Now that I am used to them they are hardly any more hassle than using paper towels. If the fabric is clean and it's just my husband and I, they are re-used. Otherwise we throw them in the laundry hamper and I do a load once a week.

When I first started using cloth napkins I would iron them straight from the washing machine while they were still damp, hang them on a drying rack then fold them a few hours later. I have refined my method and now do not iron them at all. I flick the napkins before hanging out and fold them straight from the line, smoothing out wrinkles with my hands. Freshly washed napkins go to the bottom of the pile in the kitchen drawer to rotate their use, and by the time it comes around to their turn again: *et voila*, they are pressed – albeit with a slightly insouciant air.

It was quite freeing when I decided to no longer iron my dinner napkins. I am all about removing obstacles to living the life I want. If I can find a shortcut that doesn't diminish the quality too much, I'm all over it.

I was cheered on with my ~~laziness~~ efficiency by noticing in a Ralph Lauren advertisement that the denim-blue linen napkins were *not* crisply pressed at the *très* stylish outdoor picnic setting, but rather folded and slightly rumpled.

You might think you have foods which are too messy (such as meals eaten with the fingers) or your children will wreck them, but you don't have to use the traditional starched white damask: there are many other options. Some of my favourites are made of patterned fabrics, and even the off-white twill napkins I have can survive a messy meal after a hot wash.

Introduce new traditions to your home

If you don't currently use cloth napkins at all, your family may wonder, *Why so fancy?* I know my husband did when I first put them on the dinner table. He would try not to use his napkin at all and leave it aside to save it for another night. Over time we both became more comfortable using them every day.

We do have 'good' napkins and daily-use napkins though. I was given a beautiful set made of cream linen with a monogrammed corner, and there is also a cream Indian cotton set which used to be our best dinner party set. Now that we have our monogrammed napkins, the plain set was downgraded to daily-use and our old everyday napkins went into the cleaning rag basket.

It's nice to have a good supply of cloth napkins so that you can save them up for a hot soak wash with dish towels, but if you don't want to buy a ton at once, just start with a few. I bought them whenever I saw a good deal (and I had to like the fabric and size of them of course). I prefer over-sized, so I look out for those now.

I also made a few pairs from fine cotton fabric I already had. They are a great sewing project for a beginner or anyone really, and help use up lovely fabric that you adore but don't know what to do with (I know I'm not the only one). They are good practice for measuring a square and hemming neatly.

You could even cut squares of fabric with pinking shears which creates a zig-zag edge or cut with normal scissors and then pull threads off all four sides to create a fringe – no hemming necessary.

There are so many reasons why I love dining with cloth napkins; here are just a few of my favourites:

- It's quite a green thing to do – you are not throwing paper towels away all the time.

- You will likely save money – yes, you have to buy (or make) them in the first place and wash them too, but you only have to buy cloth napkins once. Compare this to purchasing paper towels every week.

- You will feel more like the sophisticated woman you know are with a cloth napkin across your lap.

- They feel more elegant to touch than a paper towel.

- Your table will look nicer with a coloured, patterned or off-white napkin than paper towels.

- You can have different colours and fabrics to accent your décor and suit your mood.

- Seasonal napkins are a nice touch – personally I don't have seasonal napkins, but I do sometimes have a food/napkin match: I made a pair from blue and white fabric which has a Mediterranean feeling and I often use these when serving pasta.

- They help you eat better and more elegantly. We eat fewer takeaways than we used to, and when we do buy something, I serve up on ceramic plates rather than eat from the container. Cloth napkins help elevate everything.

When I think of the way I want to live, I often ask myself what an elegant five-star hotel would do. Would they use paper towels? Non!

You are beautifying your entire family's experience

We don't have children, but I think if we did, dining with cloth napkins on an everyday basis would help them learn how to comport themselves at the table.

Along the same lines it is nicer to eat with a tablecloth or placemats and real plates and cutlery (flatware). Basically, nothing disposable. If you are used to disposable table supplies, it may feel like such a hassle to start using items you have to wash and take care of, but there are benefits to this way of living. You will take ownership of your possessions and pride in your home.

When I've taken the time to look after the things I own, it feels good. When I clean, mend if needed (I'm talking more about clothes here, I don't save chipped plates or glasses) and generally take care of my possessions, I appreciate them more. This in turn helps me feel grateful that I have a cozy home which shelters us from the world.

Use your good things today

You may already have cloth napkins that are at the bottom of a kitchen or dining room drawer, languishing away never being put into service. If this is the case, why not use them tonight? See how different it feels and what your family says. Don't be surprised if they pull back and look at you with a, 'Whoa, what's this?' look on their faces. They may ask you if the queen is coming for dinner.

Don't worry if you think they will get dirty and be ruined. Without taking things to a ridiculous level, I honestly would rather use everything I own at the risk of breaking it or getting it too dirty to be saved. What's the alternative? Having cupboards full of saved 'good' stuff and using only the old or disposable items?

I used to be like that and it didn't change overnight, but one day I realized I might as well not have the nice things if they were never to be used. From then on I started serving up on good plates, sipping from fine glassware and using cloth napkins.

At first, it felt decadent and a little bit naughty; like I was using my parents' fancy items when they weren't home. In the many years since I made this decision, we might have lost a few glasses and the odd plate from breakages, but for the most part we still have everything we did. It's just that we now enjoy them.

Using the cloth napkins already in your kitchen drawer is one step towards living more elegantly every day. Why save elegance for a special occasion? Isn't every day we are breathing on this good earth a special occasion?

Make the decision once, and then it's just what you do

By building automatic habits into your day such as setting the table with a cloth napkin, knife and fork before you serve up dinner (even if it's a curry that you picked up on the way home), it gives you pause to appreciate a little bit of civility and the ability to enjoy your meal in a more mindful way.

In addition, if you know you have a cloth napkin on your lap, subconsciously you may eat more neatly because you don't want to dirty the fabric. With paper towels you can dive in with your hands and not worry that food is around your mouth. But do you really want this 'freedom'?

Then, when you need to, run a hot wash with all your napkins, tea towels and dish cloths. We don't have a clothes drier, so I hang them on the line outside (or a drying rack inside if it's raining), and it is so nice to fold them neatly once they are dry. It doesn't take long and there is something satisfying about restoring order to a small heap of crumpled napkins off the line.

If you want to wash them with the towels and throw them in the drier, that's good too. I'm all for anything that makes life easier and I try not to feel guilty or like I 'should' do something differently.

Start with one small change today, maybe it's using those cloth napkins, and see how nice it feels.

Thirty Chic Days inspirational ideas:

Train yourself into new habits. Think back to how you ate as a child with your parents. Were you taught good habits, or have you had to train yourself? Imagine how people you admire might eat and look at a few simple ways you can emulate them.

Make changes slowly. My husband is always keen to watch television with dinner, but every so often I set the table and we light a candle and chat together while we dine. You may experience a kickback from your family if you try to change everything at once and go from takeaways and paper towels in front of the television to eating at the table with cloth dinner napkins and classical music playing, so take it slow. Introduce small changes one at a time.

Writing this chapter has inspired me to have a dig through my small fabric stash and make a set of new napkins for myself. What about you? What are your takeaways from this chapter?

Day 16

Be the happiest person you know

I haven't always been seduced by the charms of positive thinking, but these days I believe having a sunny outlook is the secret of youth and happiness.

Yes, it might sound hokey, and being called a Pollyanna is rarely a compliment, but think about the people you know. Who are the ones you are always happiest to hear from? Is it the folk who usually have a smile on their face and a new interest to tell you about? Or is it the perpetual moaners who will immediately update you on what's going badly in their life, or failing that, the latest tragedies in the news. Exactly. I'd go for the Pollyanna any time.

And please don't think I am an uncaring person who won't be around when something goes horribly wrong for you. I will always be there in a crisis, but some people go through life only noticing the bad things and dismissing the good. That's the kind of learned habit of negativity I am talking about.

Still, it's easy to forget about that being-positive-thing when you're in a grump. When you can't be bothered with life. When you notice every little nit-picky thing that is annoying you *right now*.

When you feel like that, it's convenient to forget what you look like from the outside. It's easy to see when someone else is behaving badly, but not so simple to pick up when that someone is *you*. I say all this from prior experience because I can be a royal pain in the derriere, and I am grateful that my husband is a tolerant and low-drama man who chooses to overlook my less fine moments.

Still, God loves a tryer, and so I try and try again to cultivate and maintain my positivity. The good news is that it becomes more habitual the more you do it, or so I have found. But beware... the same is true of negativity. If I catch myself watching the news too often or indulging in gossip and cynicism, my formerly sunny outlook can quickly spiral downwards.

Always have things that excite you

One sure-fire way to feel buoyant about your life and therefore exude good vibes, is always to have something to be excited about – an interest or focus. It might be a good book, craft project, fitness goal or you are contemplating adopting a pet.

I love writing, and never feel better than when I start on a new book project. I enjoy deciding the topic, mapping out my chapters and then getting down to work and writing each section.

Excitement creates momentum, so find something you are enthused about and start with an action – no matter how small – towards it.

It might not be adding new things to your life – maybe you are subtracting. Decluttering your whole home may sound like an overwhelming job, but by starting small with one room, closet or category, you will soon feel the benefits and transformation that such a project provides.

If my siblings and I ever complained we were bored, our mother always told us 'bored people are boring' and sent us off to find something to do. All three of us have constant projects on the go now, so her ~~nagging~~ wise advice worked.

To always have something of interest in my life, I keep a running list of books I'd like to read, craft projects I want to make, meal ideas to try and fun 'homework' I want to complete (such as the various e-Courses or self-development books I have purchased over the years). I have health goals and love to create my dream lifestyle visions for the future too.

Having lists such as these gives me a sense of anticipation. I love having things to look forward to and it's a good day when I've done my jobs and can choose something off my 'exciting projects' list to start with.

Be the person who talks about ideas

There is a great saying which goes:

'Big people talk about ideas; small people talk about other people.'

It is a shortened form of the Eleanor Roosevelt quote:

'Great minds discuss ideas; average minds discuss events (or things); small minds discuss people.'

When I heard these sayings I immediately loved them, even though they poked at me in a rather uncomfortable way, because I have been that person who has talked about other people many times.

Gossiping feels yucky and can often lead to feeling superior or inferior (and neither are good feelings). Talking about an object or event is fairly interesting (depending on the object or event) but talking about an idea with someone is often fun and invigorating. It can also spark off new ideas of your own.

When the conversation has turned, or been steered, to ideas, I've found I have had highly interesting talks with friends and family about things I never knew they were interested in.

Asking open-ended questions along the lines of:

What would you really like to do if you could choose anything?

What would you do for a job if you could live your dream life?

Would you live in a different country if it was easy and you had an amazing job to go to? What country? What job?

You don't need to go into a social situation prepared with an official list of questions (wouldn't that be geeky!), but you can steer the conversation towards interesting waters by noticing when someone mentions something and then ask them, 'Can you tell me more about that?' or 'Wow, so interesting, tell me more'.

I have found that some variation of 'tell me more' is a phrase which leads to extremely satisfying conversations.

Cultivate happiness as a daily habit

Since I started choosing to look at the positive as a matter of course, so much has changed for me. I almost feel like my good fortune has come from nowhere, but I know it is because of choices I have made and daily actions I take.

About three years ago my husband and I had an amazing talk where we decided that we wanted to shake our life up. It was spurred on by our retail business lease coming up for renewal and we started thinking about whether we wanted to continue with this work. If we decided to sell the business we were free to live anywhere, so we also talked about whether we wanted to continue living in the same area. In the end we decided to sell our business and home to move away from the city, to the small provincial area where I'd grown up.

That decision led to where we are today: living on a peaceful semi-rural four-acre property with our pets. I write my books from my home office and my husband has a new job that he loves. Our life is low-key and low-stress, and it's all because we chose for it to be that way.

People say how lucky we are and I do feel extremely lucky. Every day one of us will look at each other and say, 'We actually live here' and 'How lucky are we?'

I truly believe it all comes down to positive thoughts which led to positive actions, and also by trusting that we would be okay in the future no matter what. The old me was quite distrustful and you can tell it's a negative attribute to have.

I know that our future will only get better and better, and I want to tell people what I took years to figure out for myself: When you think you are being 'realistic', you are being negative. I used to think being realistic was being honest, and that cynicism meant you would never be ripped off. I am still a careful person and wouldn't call myself gullible, but so much has changed for me since I decided to become the most positive person I know.

It's something I am still working on, but as long as I am more positive than not, I am happy. No-one is perfect, and there are always new areas I come across which show I am not being my most positive self. I love finding them because then I can upgrade them.

I try to be a pleasure to be around and enjoy finding conversation topics which light other people up. When I am asked a question, I quickly think about my first response before I share it – does it have a happy feel to it? I also smile more often, which is not only pleasant for others, but makes me feel happier too. Have you noticed when someone smiles at you that their entire face changes? It's like a light has been switched on.

The same goes for the words you speak. When you focus on the good, it is nicer for whoever is listening to you, plus it is excellent for your mental health to not dwell on everything that has annoyed you that day. If there are things that have gone wrong, fix them up or forget about them. Dwell in the beauty of your day instead.

Please don't dismiss positivity as a fake and unnecessary thing. It will make everything in your life better, I promise you. Bad times will seem more manageable and good times will blow your mind. Come on, jump on the bandwagon!

Thirty Chic Days inspirational ideas:

Consider how you sound to others. Choose your words and topics carefully, and note when you enjoy talking to someone; what was it about them? The way they spoke? What they said? The way they smiled every so often as they talked? Perhaps it was their sparky energy. How can you cultivate what you noticed for yourself?

Decide that every decision you make will be the right one, even when you might not be so sure at the time. Definitely make informed decisions, don't rush into something parroting 'It will all be okay!', but don't second-guess yourself either. When you go into anything with an air of 'I've made a good decision', you have.

Things might twist and turn on you, but in the end you will see that whatever happened was for your highest good. Try it for yourself: look back at something you chose that didn't quite work out like you planned; I'm sure you could say that something *even better* came along instead. Or at the very least, you learned a valuable lesson which has served you well.

When I think about my first marriage which ended in divorce, I sometimes wonder if it would have been better if we weren't married, and simply dated for a few years before splitting up. Then I decided that I might have met someone who was okay for me but not great, and we would have stayed together forever.

I met my second husband, and love of my life at 32. If I had met someone who was 'good enough', I wouldn't have married the person who is perfect for me. Life always works out, just sometimes in unexpected ways.

Be your own cheerleader. When you are doing something; maybe it's prepping the ingredients for your family's dinner or finishing up, cheer yourself on. 'Yay, Fiona! Well done! Go you!' Of course, you will use your own name, not mine...

By surrounding yourself with positivity in lots of little ways you will slowly brainwash yourself over time. I often do this for myself, either out loud or in my head, and it's a little thing but all those little things add up. I always get a shock when I am talking with someone I haven't seen for a while, or even a complete stranger, and they are extremely negative. It stands out so clearly to me now, but I used to be like that.

I have since realized that a common denominator of successful people is that they are positive, can-do go-getters who are always cheering themselves – and others – on. A wealthy and elegant friend of mine who is always such good company when we meet for coffee once said, 'I love to hear of others doing well' when I was telling her about someone I knew.

Why not take on this way of thinking and give yourself the best chance of success in all areas of your amazing life?

Day 17
Create your own chic manifesto

Perhaps, like me, you've read a million books, blogs and articles on living a chic lifestyle. There is so much of interest out there that you can't help yourself. It can almost become like a treasure hunt where you think the next Kindle book or online resource will hold the gold you seek.

Instead of bringing you closer to your idealistic way of living though, you find yourself feeling further away than ever from your glittering future chic life. You feel overwhelmed because there is so much goodness to take in.

When I first started my 'chic journey' it was new and exciting, and I devoured everything I could find on the topic. After a while though, I found that when I had too many external influences and other people's voices in my head, I became cloudy on what *I* wanted. I was filled up with ideas!

For some of us it's a cyclical thing where sometimes we're happy taking in more of other people's opinions and at other times less. We become 'full' and we don't need anything more for a while.

Happily, it doesn't take long to get my own thoughts back and feel in balance again. Something that helps me feel surer of the direction I'm going in (while still being inspired by others), is to note down **my own take on being chic**.

I sat down and came up with my top ten timeless chic principles to guide me – my own chic manifesto if you will. How fancy and official does that sound? It was such a fun project, and a real mind-expander to think about too. Here it is:

{Fiona's Chic Manifesto - my ten chic principles}

Chic principle 1: I love what I love

I am me, no matter who I am around. Because I love all things chic, I will not dull myself down to fit in with others. I will delight in pretty details in my home and personal style regardless of what's in fashion or what others may think. I dress in a way that makes me feel happy and inspired.

Chic principle 2: I please myself

I share as much or as little as I am comfortable sharing. Others will not pressure me into giving away more than I want to. I enjoy having mystique and moving freely through life in my own cloak of mystery. I don't feel the need to explain myself and am happy to live my life without commentary.

Chic principle 3: I am a queen
I treat myself with exquisite care. I love my body because she is my vessel in this life. I take care of her by feeding her nourishing foods, pampering her with self-care and giving her adequate rest. I listen to what she tells me. I appreciate, accept and love her exactly as she is.

Chic principle 4: I am kind
I treat others with compassion and empathy. Everyone is doing the best they can, and most people are kind. I try and see things from their point of view and it makes it easy to be the type of person I want to be. I am gentle and soft in my approach towards others.

Chic principle 5: I am savvy
I am a good steward of my resources. I appreciate my income and all the possessions I have been blessed with. Anything I don't need any more is donated so that someone else can make use of it and I can enjoy the space in my life. I am grateful for everything I have and all that is to come.

Chic principle 6: I am abundant

I am ambitious for a wonderful, fabulous, sparkling and magical life and it begins today. I am constantly dreaming up new and better ways to make my life more fun and happy. In turn that cheer spills over to others, and as I become more prosperous I can help better the causes close to my heart.

Chic principle 7: I am creative

I am inspired by the latest fashions each season and how others put their style together, and at the same time enjoy dressing uniquely in a way that reflects the spirit of the true me. I purchase and wear only that which makes my heart sing and I am grateful for a wardrobe that lifts me up every single day.

Chic principle 8: I matter

Even though I may sometimes feel small or insignificant, I know I am a valuable member of the human race and have a lot to contribute to my circle of influence. This includes my family, friends, acquaintances, online friends and readers – everyone I come into contact with. I take on this responsibility.

Chic principle 9: I create my own sanctuary

I enjoy my home and appreciate how lucky I am to live in a safe country with a warm and cozy place to shelter. I show this appreciation by keeping my home clutter-free, tidy and clean. I support my home and it supports me.

Chic principle 10: I am inspired
I am constantly inspired by both myself and others. I welcome the ideas I dream up and am thankful that we are able to gain – and share – inspiration and wisdom from – and with – others around us.

~~

When I wrote this manifesto, what helped was thinking about everything that made me feel empowered and hopeful. Sometimes when you have that overwhelmed feeling, you can feel anything but. Then, re-reading through my manifesto from time to time helps me remember that I am responsible for my own fabulous destiny.

Benefits of having a chic manifesto

Perhaps you feel inspired to create your own personal manifesto. I'd definitely recommend it as a fun and inspiring exercise which will uplift you in the following ways:

You will easily zero in on what you value
You will feel empowered that you can shape your life
You will feel effortlessly inspired
You are less likely to self-sabotage
You will feel happier because you are in control
You will appreciate YOU more instead of thinking others have it better

You will enjoy the simple pleasures of life
You will no longer desire to accumulate more, more, more
Your self-esteem will rise
You will have your own guidance to follow

These are all ways in which writing my personal 'chic' manifesto has helped me. It aided me in working out what was important to me. And because it is a relatively short document, I can read it often to assist me in remembering how I want to be. It is a constant source of inspiration for how I want to live my life. And yes, it strengthens and empowers me, and it does give me hope.

Can you imagine how reading your personal manifesto every morning might set up your day to go well? Even if some days it doesn't feel as impactful as others, your wise words will still sink in.

It doesn't need to be set in stone either. You might change words or phrases from time to time, or feel like creating a completely new manifesto for, say, the new year, your birthday, or a new beginning such as getting married (or divorced), having a child or moving into the empty nest phase of your life.

If you need more inspiration, simply Google 'chic personal manifesto' or 'personal manifesto' and look at the Images, or search on Pinterest. I love doing this because it's fun to read others' manifestos. Many of them are beautifully designed and have points that inspire me to add to my manifesto.

In my research while writing this chapter, I saw that some personal manifestos are simply a list of words. For me that would include my 'value' words such as:

Freedom
Peace
Creativity

You can create a mini-manifesto for a certain part of your life that you'd like to focus on too. It might be a fashion and style manifesto, a healthy body manifesto or a manifesto for your home.

It's so fun to create your own inspiration and I hope this chapter has inspired you to consider designing a personal manifesto for yourself.

Thirty Chic Days inspirational ideas:

Have a think about **what might belong on *your* manifesto**. To best work that out, write down:

- Things that are important to you – people, values, ways of being
- Things that overwhelm you, then take the opposite of them as a goal
- Attributes of those you admire, whether in real life or public figures

Then start **letting words and ideas** form in your mind.

If it seems like a big project, **start with a mini-manifesto** to warm up your creativity.

However you start, **let your words be fanciful and dreamy**. If phrases pop into your mind, write them down. This is your own personal space to craft your beautiful life.

Have fun with it!

Day 18
Embrace your inner bombshell

There is the elegant part of my personality who loves classical music, Chanel No. 5, French subtitled movies and dressing in a casual/classic/Paris chic style.

And then there is the *other* side of me. She loves watching the Real Housewives of Beverly Hills, wearing the latest celebrity fragrance, surrounding herself with sparkly things, and has an hourglass figure which is definitely *not* Paris skinny.

I have always felt like this side of me was *too much*. That I should try harder to be more demure, less bossy and outspoken, not have such big boobs, not be too loud and too... *me*.

I'd compare myself to naturally slim girls with stylish small busts who could wear anything, thinking, 'I should try harder to be that skinny, I shouldn't enjoy food so much, I should play it cool more, I shouldn't be so enthusiastic'. It was exhausting!

I tried to tamp down this side of me and hope she'd go away. But I also felt like life would be *so* deathly boring without her by my side. She gave me spice and fun and *happiness*. So I kept her my secret pleasure, occasionally letting a little bit of her out on my blog, but mostly keeping her hidden and indulging her whims at home.

I thought if I let her run the show I could no longer have a blog called *How to be Chic*; I mean, the two sides are incompatible, aren't they? It felt like this internal struggle against my desire to be the perfect French-styled girl, and my natural essence who is... *the bombshell.*

I realized this relatively recently, that this side of me was a bombshell. As soon as the word popped into my mind, it felt good; it felt like me.

The more I thought about it, the more I realized that I had been denying my inner bombshell when all she wanted to do was be my friend. Looking at pins saved on my Pinterest boards, there was a lot of bombshell there. Mind you, these were all on my secret boards, the boards that I didn't want anyone to see. Only chic and elegant pins were allowed on my public Pinterest boards!

I think this is something I have been pushing down my entire life because it's too much, too sexy and too unsafe. As a girl growing up I'm sure I was shaped by those around me; to be a good girl, not show off too much, not bare too much skin and don't be too loud.

Making the decision to follow my inner bombshell bliss feels like I am allowing myself to blossom, take ownership of my happiness and stop apologizing for my big boobs and my fun-loving tacky side.

The bombshell is feminine whilst still being a powerhouse, and I love that. She is out and out woman. I like a blend of the old-school and the modern bombshell too, from Marilyn Monroe to Erika Jayne.

To crystalize my own take on the bombshell, I started brainstorming a list to work out what bombshell means to me and what place she will take in my life, because my bombshell isn't a burlesque dancer or about to start dressing like Peggy Bundy. No, my bombshell is a misty rose-tinted vision of femininity, strength, passion and *fabulousness*.

Essence of bombshell a la Fiona

Rose gold
Long hot showers
Moisturized soft and fragrant skin
Hair that smells good
Light, luminous and golden makeup
Sexy fit and glowy - just been for a run
Real Housewives of Beverly Hills
Kim Kardashian
Beauty rituals
Face masks

Early nights
A glass of champagne
Billie Holiday/Sarah Vaughan/Ella Fitzgerald
Lullaby in Birdland
Hotel lobby piano music
Kind, sweet-natured and playful
Silky and sensual loungewear
Getting lost in a book
Old school beauty regimen: tissue-off cleanser, Olay facial lotion, lathering with Lux soap
Boudoir time
A beautiful bathroom
Good posture – shoulders back and chest out
Happy confidence
She likes herself

So much goodness started happening inside of me when I embraced my inner bombshell instead of turning her away. I had inadvertently popped the lid off something big and was positively buzzing!

My clothing style started to evolve as well. I still love denim and casual chic, but I immediately started wearing more form-fitting tops. I had been buying a size bigger, so they wouldn't be so tight across my bust, but then there was more fabric around the torso and it ended up looking dowdy and frumpy; but hey, at least I couldn't be accused of flaunting a big bust right?

I started tailoring a few of my clothing pieces such as tops and dresses, by curving in the side seams so that they were a bit more fitted around my waist. This has worked well because I have quite broad shoulders and back width, so the tops fit well there, then they will taper in under my bra line which flatters my shape more.

I have been taking the time to put a little bit of makeup on each day too (rather than rush it or skip makeup altogether) and let my hair dry in waves. Because of the low humidity where we live, I can let my hair air-dry in the summer and it looks pretty. It's my natural look and it's also better for my hair not to have heat used on it all the time.

I have been doing my nails – my current preferred style is quite short and painted in a dark or bright shade (with a creamy finish – no sparkle or shimmer).

I have been wearing my wedges and heels more often, even if just out for lunch or to the supermarket with my husband. Wearing them for short bursts of time is fine for comfort, and I feel sexier. Why not wear them more often? My husband always says how nice I look whenever I wear them too. I still wear Birkenstocks and jandals (flip flops/thongs) around the house, but it feels good to wear my heels, because, well, I'm a bombshell.

To those around me, I probably haven't changed that much. The alterations to my clothes are subtle, and I already wore heels sometimes too. It's more an inner seismic shift where I feel better about myself and no longer have shame for my bombshell side.

It seems strange that finding the right word has changed everything for me, but it has. Having love and acceptance towards myself has always been something I've struggled with, even with all the mantras and personal development work.

It felt like the last puzzle piece had fallen into place, or at least enough of the puzzle to be able to see what the picture really was. It was as if up until then I was trying to fit some pieces in from a different puzzle. It felt muddied and like it was hard work to create my most ideal self, but I wasn't about to stop trying.

Now I feel like I can relax and still be a success. I can be me – the bombshell! Now when I look in the mirror and say 'I love you Fiona' like I've always tried to do (a la Louise Hay), it feels like I believe it. Can you relate to this? If not your inner bombshell, what side of you are you denying?

An unexpected side benefit is that my appetite for sweet foods (which was the bane of my life) has fallen away. I haven't been thinking about it or craving them as much.

It's almost like a pulled muscle that ends up affecting other muscles around it because they are compensating for that muscle. By denying this side of me that I didn't think measured up to my chic ideal, I was creating all sorts of havoc in my mind. Isn't the human psyche *so* fascinating?

I hope this chapter inspires you to have a think about the things you do that you're ashamed of. Think of all those habits you wish you didn't have. Do they have a common theme?

Look at words and see if you can find one that fits you as well as *bombshell* does for me. Other words that I tried on such as *goddess* did not fit so well. They were close but not quite there. Perhaps it is bombshell or goddess for you, or perhaps it's something else altogether.

I implore you to let this side of you speak out, because she's dying to share all her inspiration with you. Good luck!

Thirty Chic Days inspirational ideas:

What gives your life spice? Write down all the things that light you up even though you feel like they shouldn't because they're not how you imagine yourself. What are those television programs you love, books you read and fashion looks you are drawn to that you think 'I shouldn't like that, it's too tacky/loud/not me, etc'?

Brainstorm and find what feels like YOU. Write down as many words as possible to uncover their ideas and essence. Is there a word in there that jumps out at you? When I fell upon *bombshell*, it was like a lightbulb went off. Suddenly everything made sense and all my disparate loves that I tried so hard to squash down knitted together beautifully. What is that word for you?

As you go through this process of discovery, make a list of everything you love, such as I have done above. What picture can you see emerging?

Have fun while you're doing it. I invite you to look upon this chapter as getting to know yourself even more than you already do.

Love and accept every part of yourself, even (especially) the parts that make you cringe a little bit. For me those bits are when I get excited and talk too much, when I see my giant bust in a mirror when I'm out shopping and when I spritz on the latest celebrity fragrance even though I 'should' choose something more stylish.

Own that side of yourself; better than that, embrace her. She is part of you too and she will ensure that you have a good time, and isn't that what life's all about? Time is too precious not to live *la vie d'une bombe* (the life of a bombshell) or whatever your own divine inner essence is.

Day 19
Don't talk, just do

I had a truth-telling thought come to me recently, and it said, 'the more you talk about something, the less you feel like doing it'. Hearing this felt like a lightning bolt even though I am familiar with the concept.

I mention something similar in a chapter of my first *Thirty Chic Days* book: '*Day 5 – Create and guard your secret garden*' where I recommend *not* sharing new thoughts and ideas with other people straight away. Not only could they pour cold water on them, but also because letting out your exciting idea could leak some of the energy of it. Both of these things can cause your enthusiasm to wane and the plan goes nowhere.

A few examples of this type of situation come to mind:

When I want to eat healthier

After a period of letting loose a little and eating more potato chips and chocolate than I normally do – often at Christmas, but also at other times of the year – I will decide to cut back on treat foods and amp up the nutrition of my three daily meals. Rather than enlisting my husband's help and announcing my plan to him, I find it far better for me to follow my own little steps as follows:

One. Inspire myself with photos of myself when slimmer, and online images of slender celebrities and public figures I admire. Also, I peruse my inspiration files where I have saved articles and snippets of slimming motivation, as well as affirmations I have written for myself.

Two. Let this fuel my motivation to skip after-lunch sweet treats and pre-dinner snacks and feel empowered by these actions, not deprived. I happily sip water all day, order the small size if I am eating out, and choose more nutritious options.

Three. Keep in mind the vision of me not only fitting, but looking amazing wearing anything from my wardrobe. Organize my closet and revisit the pieces I want to wear again, and feel excited for that day.

Four. Don't succumb to the enticing 'strict diet' habit

of old. Strictness never works for me – I immediately rebel against myself. I just need to keep on with my daily self-encouragement and motivation and know that I will be slipping into my smaller-size clothes one day soon.

This is how I make 'dieting' fun and easy, and it's highly motivating to me. I don't cut out all treats, but I do manage my 'fun' binges and refrain from buying foods that I know will set me off.

Others may have a completely different way of approaching weight loss however. My husband goes about it in a masculine and linear way (naturally, since he is a man), and is strict until he is at the weight he wants to be, without deviating for even a mouthful. I know that doesn't work for me, so I do my own thing, by myself.

My husband only wants the best for me and he would help me in any way he could, but he isn't female, and he isn't me. That's why his helpful advice about what works for him is best avoided by keeping my mouth zipped while I steer myself back towards a healthier lifestyle.

Everyday tasks

Sometimes on a weekend day I'll say, 'I'm going to have a shower now', only to be pottering around in my nightshirt an hour or two later. I also faux-complain about the cats cluttering our bed so that it will be hard to make it. I comment on all the fur I have to vacuum from our duvet cover and how there are paw prints on the white linen.

When I have *not* gone on and on about these things, I just do them. Talking about these tasks seems to lessen my motivation, not encourage it as I previously thought. And, how boring would it be for the person I live with to hear my inane chatter?

When I've found myself showering at lunchtime instead of mid-morning (mid-morning is pretty good on a Sunday? Isn't it?) or making the bed at 3pm (also on a Sunday...) I can't help but think to myself 'If I would *do* something rather than just talk about it, it would have been completed hours ago and I could be doing something more enjoyable'.

It's a shame that talking about something doesn't get that job done, isn't it?

Exciting projects you've always wanted to do

But what about a big project, such as writing a book, completing a quilt or learning an instrument or foreign language. Do we talk endlessly about what we'd like to do and never quite get around to doing it? Yes! I've done this so many times, yet if I'd just shut my mouth and make plans and action steps to get on with it, I'd have completed everything on my wish list by now.

Yes, I have broken the seal on writing books and this is my sixth one, so I can feel proud of that (It's not that hard! Write for half-an-hour a day to start with and gain momentum – you can do it!); but I also have many projects I have talked about for years, decades maybe, and I'm always saying, 'I'm going to make a big denim quilt out of all the jeans I've saved up' (I know it will look better than it sounds!).

But have I even started it? Heck no. And I am slowly eating up my worn-out jean stash making cushion covers, place mats and coasters. The thing to consider here is that perhaps I didn't really want to make a quilt, but my blah-blah-blah mouth hadn't quite caught up with my brain.

And here is where it all ties back in neatly to the title of this chapter: Don't talk, just do'. I have achieved *so much* more in terms of all my projects – writing, organizing my closet, being slim and healthy, sewing, cooking, home ideas etc – because I don't endlessly talk about them anymore, I just do them.

Of course, I'll talk about them a little bit, especially to someone else involved such as my husband with our home décor, but as for the rest, it feels far better to keep my ideas inside as I incubate them. I made this quote up for myself a while back and wrote it on an index card. It goes:

'A self-possessed woman radiates from the inside. Keep your secret garden private and its energy will be harnessed to power you elegantly from within.'

I read this to remind myself of this wisdom, because I truly forget it, all the time. Then a little thought bubble pops into my mind as in the first paragraph of this chapter – 'The more I talk about doing something, the less I feel like doing it' and it's as if I've heard that concept for the first time.

I feel like a goldfish with their (supposed) two-second memory, having 'new' (old) revelations all the time. Oh well, better than not getting those rehashed revelations at all right, right?

The difference between men and women

Women talk more than men as a rule. I saw a statistic on bbc.com that says women speak 20,000 words per day and men speak 7,000... No wonder they tune out; I know my husband does, he can't help it.

He is a good, caring and kind person and loves me to the moon and back, but, I talk a lot. Gosh, I even get sick of myself sometimes when I hear myself going blah blah blah and I stop, sometimes even in the middle of a sentence and just. shut. up. Funnily enough, my husband doesn't even react because he hasn't noticed I didn't finish my stream of consciousness thought. That's when you know it's bad!

All is not lost though, and it's not like I am changing some innate part of myself to please him. Blathering on and on about complaints or my endless writing plans isn't fun for either of us. For him, poor guy, having to listen to it, and for me, I don't want to perpetuate unpleasantness by going on about bad service or someone rude; and I also don't want to let out all the good energy which is powering my exciting ideas.

Don't talk, just do; it's my new life motto (or one of them anyway). Won't you join me? Let's see what we can achieve together.

Thirty Chic Days inspirational ideas:

Think about all the times **you've spilled your soul** in a big excited gush to someone who didn't match your enthusiasm, or worse, started pointing out all the reasons why your plan couldn't work.

Instead, next time you get an exciting idea to try, **keep it to yourself**. The secret nature of your plan will feel so big that you will find yourself effortlessly motivated to write 500 words a day; swap the afternoon super-duper-mocha-locha-cino for a chic black coffee; or start your weekly meal planning project.

Be one of those ladies where people notice, 'hey, you look great, have you lost weight?' or 'your outfit looks amazing!' or 'I can't believe you come up with so many great meal ideas'. These comments are quite a thrill when it's something you've been working on.

You might share your secret with them if you think they will appreciate it, or you might simply say 'thank you for noticing' and **slip your cloak of elegant mystique** around your shoulders.

Day 20
Have a daily success plan

When my husband and I sold our retail footwear business at the end of 2016 and I finally had the chance to be a work-from-home writer, I quickly realized that I had to create some sort of schedule for myself.

In the hazy dreamy days of my ideal future, I pictured myself effortlessly gliding through the day; writing, exercising, making delicious meals, pottering and organizing... but the reality was quite different.

When you work in a job (or your own business like we had), the structure is already there. When you have a boss you are told what time you need to show up. Our store was open certain hours, so we had that structure to our week.

When you are at home full-time, whether it's working for yourself, being with your children or maybe you've just retired, it is up to you how your day looks. This is an exciting prospect, but strangely can feel quite unsettling.

When I worked full-time, I had practice runs on my days off, but it wasn't so important then. I could have a day noodling about, doing a few jobs and relaxing too; but because I knew I had to be back at work the next day it focused my mind.

Having *every* day available to me took that structure away. If I didn't do something today, I still had tomorrow. There was no urgency to do anything so the things I didn't like as much were consistently put off, until there was a crisis point sometimes. A mini crisis point yes, but it didn't do a lot for my serenity.

Some days under my new non-schedule went well and I achieved a lot, but other days were a disaster. On those days I procrastinated most of the day and didn't get any of my jobs done let alone any of the things I told myself I wanted to do such as writing, sewing, decluttering, organizing or reading a book.

Because I hadn't done my jobs and my work, I told myself I couldn't do the fun activities. But I was procrastinating on my jobs and my work, so *nothing* got done and I didn't get to do anything enjoyable either. So silly!

Set yourself up for success

After thinking about it for a bit, I saw that it could be constructive to draw up a plan which would help me feel like I'd had a successful day. I've tried to-do lists but they didn't always work for me. I'd start writing down a few things I wanted to do the next day, but then keep adding to it as I thought of new items. Before long, the list was a daunting length. Overwhelmed, I would choose the easiest looking jobs and tick those off, ignoring the more important but less fun tasks. I love the *idea* of to-do lists, but I've found that I am a slippery character and cannot be trusted to prioritize. I needed to try another way.

How I turned it around was that I decided to create an ideal work-from-home day for myself, as if I was mapping out a schedule for an employee as their manager. The difference was that as well as my jobs and work, I'd add some fun things to do as well.

I would include prep-work for meals so that I had healthy and delicious food ready ahead of time, and plan to be finished when my husband returned home from work so that we could relax together and catch up on our respective days.

If, like me, you find to-do lists tough to stick to, maybe writing a daily success plan will work better for you as well.

Here is one of my first daily success plans that I mocked up the night before. I went into detail, even writing down my lunch menu, so that I could simply follow along, no decision-making necessary. I don't need to tell you that this day was a roaring success, and I put it all down to having my success plan ready.

My daily success plan:

6 a.m.
Get up
Put laundry on line
Hot tea and write

7 a.m.
Have breakfast and read
Tidy kitchen, empty dishwasher, tidy house, make bed
Write more, make a few calls to book appointments

10.30 a.m.
Exercise, shower, hair wash
Go to the bank

12.30 p.m.
Lunch – salad and three eggs scrambled, coffee
Watch an episode of my current favourite program
Tidy up kitchen, prep dinner, chop fruit for breakfast
Write a bit more

5.30 p.m.
My husband arrives home, we relax and catch up

7 p.m.
Dinner, kitchen tidy up
Quick house pickup

9 p.m.
Relaxing time in the bedroom, facewash, journaling
Bedtime and reading

Now that I'm in the habit of having a daily success plan, I'll usually write it out the night before, but even if I don't, all is not lost. I simply write it out as soon as I remember I haven't done it or if I find myself *drifting*, whether it is 8 a.m., 11 a.m. or even 2 p.m. I believe it's never too late to start the day or *save* the day.

When you work full-time or part-time

What about if you work outside the house though? Can you still have a daily success plan? I believe so, and in fact I wish I'd thought this idea up sooner, because I could have used it *around* my work hours as well as on my days off.

When I think about it, I probably did have a success plan most days, just not a formal one. I was always writing things down in my planner that I wanted to do different week nights after work and in the evenings. For example, I'd have a blog post planned for one night, a facemask for another and various loads of laundry spaced out during the week, so I didn't have a big pile of washing at the weekend.

You can practice a full day when you are working by making a success plan for your day off. List tasks you'd like to complete, chores to do and a few fun things as well. Then slot them into an ideal day, attaching times to certain blocks of items. I found that having a few set points in the morning and afternoon is the easiest way to stay on task.

If I had no times listed, my success plan would look like a long, daunting to-do list, but if I had a time assigned to everything, it could feel overwhelming. By having breakfast, mid-morning, lunchtime, mid-afternoon, pre-dinner and after dinner being set points, I got to slot items into areas of two to three hours.

I keep my eye on these times and it helps me focus on the tasks I said I wanted to complete, not wander off and start something that I didn't even know existed until I came across it. Thinking, 'Oh I've got all day' lures me in to start that fun-looking project and before I know it it's 3.30 p.m. and I've done nothing else.

Planning for fun and leisure

Your daily success plan doesn't always need to include chores either. Imagine if you had a day off where you planned to spend the entire day in your sewing room. This is a dream for me because I love tinkering around and sorting through my fabrics, choosing a small project to make that I can complete in one day, then finishing that project before I tidy up at dinner-time. *That* would be a successful leisure day for me.

But back to reality… here's how it really goes. I think to myself, 'I am up-to-date with laundry and the housework, and I don't have anything pressing that can't wait a day for my writing, so why don't I have a sewing day tomorrow? I can get stuck in and have a good tidy up as well as make something. What fun.'

The next day arrives and I'll get out of bed bright and early. I'll have breakfast and think, 'maybe I'll put a load of laundry through. Oh, the dishwasher needs emptying.' Then I decide to check my emails and end up browsing on my computer. Then I decide to see what we have for dinner, plus my lunch...

By this stage it's late morning and I haven't even started what I planned to. As you can imagine, the day slips away and I end up at dinner time frustrated because I haven't had my sewing session and I haven't really done many jobs either. Just where did the day go?

Imagining to myself that my sewing day was tomorrow, I might draw up a success plan that looks like this:

6 a.m.
Let the dogs out
Feed the cats
Write in bed sipping hot tea

7 a.m.
Take the dogs for a walk
Get the dogs breakfast
Have my breakfast – a NutriBullet smoothie with *everything* in it
Tidy up the kitchen

8.15 a.m.
Have a shower
Get dressed
Make the bed

9.30 a.m.
Tidy sewing room
Sort through fabrics and put them away

12 noon
Make my lunch – a microwave baked potato with leftover savoury mince and sour cream, plus a side salad
Coffee and a read
Tidy the kitchen
Prep vegetables for dinner

1.15 p.m.
Browse my file of collected sewing and craft ideas and choose something small that looks fun to make
Work on my project and complete it
Tidy up

3.30 p.m.
Tea break with a book

4 p.m.
Feed the cats and dogs
Maybe take the dogs for another little walk
Put smoothie ingredients together for the next

morning
Get dinner organized

5.30 p.m.
My husband arrives home from work
Relax outside with a drink, and chat

7 p.m.
Dinnertime
Watch a television program
Tidy kitchen
Cup of herbal tea

8.30 p.m.
Retire to the bedroom for a facemask and read Victoria magazine

9.30 p.m.
Lights out

I know that more organized people might find it hard to believe, but I find mapping out my day to be extremely helpful. I'm not sure if it's because I am a creative type, but I can find it hard to transition from one activity to another. Whatever I'm doing at that time I want to keep doing it. Having times slotted in assists me in seeing when I need to move onto something else.

They also mean that the day doesn't get away from me which has happened *so* often in the past. In addition, my success plan safeguards me against 'bright shiny object syndrome' where I see something that needs doing and start doing that, when I'd planned to do something else altogether. I used to do this all the time and it's still a tendency I have to be aware of.

Perhaps you can relate to this chapter? If you find to-do lists sometimes don't work so well for you, why not create a daily success plan instead. I think you will be pleasantly surprised, as I was, at how helpful this exercise is. It is fun to think about, easy to follow and extremely motivating. In fact, when I write out a success plan for the next day, I can't wait to go to bed so I can wake up bright and early to get started on it!

Thirty Chic Days inspirational ideas:

Start with a master list and a calendar. Your master list is where you write out everything you need and want to get done, as well as fun things you'd like to do. All chores, jobs, tasks and projects go on this list.

Your calendar will contain appointments and tasks that need to be done on a certain day.

Have these both to hand when you write out tomorrow's success plan.

Map out your ideal day. Have a think about how you would love tomorrow to look and write it out with times and details. Include both tasks and fun projects (or part of a project if it's a big one) and direct your day with some loose structure in the form of times.

Don't cram things in too tightly. Be generous with your estimation of how long things will take. This is *not* a competition of how many tasks you can get done in one day, rather it will be a relaxing and enjoyable framework for you to do some jobs, have some fun, and overall feel proud of yourself at the end of the day. You will feel fulfilled and happy with yourself, not regretful or wrung out. Sound good?

Refine as you go. If you come across a fun (or not) project to do as you go throughout your day and it's not urgent, add it to your master list so you don't forget it. Then, you are free to continue with your plan. You can complete this task on another day.

Remember, making a daily plan for yourself is most successful when you:

- Write everything down
- Attach times periodically throughout the day (link them to other things such as appointment times, ideal meal times, a television program you want to watch, people getting home from school or work, or your own job)
- Don't include too many items in one day
- Have fun things planned as well as chores
- Finish at a reasonable hour

Good luck and have fun!

Day 21
Reframe everything to be beautiful, magical and luxurious

Several months ago, I started taking a supplement called 'Beauty Oil' recommended to me by a friend. It is made by a company here in New Zealand called Bestow and has only two ingredients: cold-pressed organic flax seed and safflower oils. You can use it in smoothies, over food or as a salad dressing; but I drink one tablespoon each morning straight. It's not cheap so I don't want to waste a drop.

I'm sure it is doing magical things to my body, but what I almost love more about Beauty Oil is its name. As soon as my friend mentioned it to me I knew I had to try it, because it sounded so appealing. Oil that is going to make you beautiful!

I was pondering why I was so taken with Beauty Oil and concluded that it would not be so compelling if it was called Health Oil or even Wellbeing Oil. Beauty Oil has a luxurious touch to it, so well done to the marketing team at Bestow.

It gave me the idea to call other healthy changes I wanted to make by a different name too. For a start, beauty changes instead of healthy changes. Beauty is not a vain and shallow attribute to love. Beauty comes from health. When you see a woman walk past and think 'she's beautiful', it's often because she is glowing with good health and radiant happiness.

In this chapter you will find how I became inspired to look after myself better by replacing 'health' with 'beauty'.

Beauty food

When people clean up their diets and trade in junk food and soda for fresh fruits, vegetables and hydrating water, they will naturally become more attractive. I've seen it on television programs and in real life; also in myself.

Our bodies will look better when we feed them natural nutrients and foods they can digest well. It's a logical fact that I'm sure we all know, but it can still be hard to stick to a healthy diet.

What about beauty food or going on a beauty diet though? How lovely does that sound? I would *always* choose beauty food over the alternative if it was named thus. To me beauty food conjures up fresh fruits and vegetables, healthy fats and a moderate amount of protein with each meal. Beauty food includes many different bright colours from nature and is water-rich.

Um, does that sound like a healthy diet to you? Because it does to me too. But when I label it as beauty food rather than healthy food, I crave it more. I look forward to mealtimes so I can enhance my beauty with food.

Rather than forcing yourself to choose the healthy option over something you'd rather eat instead, beauty food attracts you to the plate and promises you a lifetime of lushness and vibrancy.

Beauty sleep

Well, how handy is that? Beauty sleep has already been so-named a long time ago. How convenient. 'I can't stay up too late, gotta get my beauty sleep.' How many times have you heard someone say that? It's a phrase which was ingrained into me when I was younger. Thankfully it's a good belief to have.

There have been so many studies done that prove when you get the right amount of good sleep, the healthier, slimmer, more productive and happier you will be.

Staying up late is a little bit like junk food for me. I think it will be fun at the time, but in the morning, I regret it. I love to go to bed between 9 p.m. and 10 p.m. and have the lights out by 10 p.m. or 10.30 p.m. at the latest. I relax in the evening and most nights will do the things that will enable me to have a good night's rest. I don't do any computer work after dinner and I try not to spend too much time scrolling on my phone.

I'll watch one television program after dinner, then read for about half an hour in bed. Reading before I go to sleep always helps me sleep well. I make sure to put my phone in flight mode too, so I'm not disturbed overnight.

We bought a new bed last year after saving up and researching the best one to get. It is huge and luxe and I do believe I sleep better on it than in our old bed.

It was quite expensive (in my mind) but when I worked out the cost for each of us if we kept it for a conservative ten years (and we'll likely keep it for fifteen at least), it works out to $325 each per year. Less than $1 a day. For the best sleep ever! I'm so glad I worked that out because it made me happier to pay such a price for a bed.

Even before we bought our new bed I made it as easy as possible for me to get a good night's sleep with soft, clean sheets, relaxing music playing quietly and a soothing wind-down time before bed, to ensure that I got my beauty sleep.

Beauty walk

It takes me a lot to love exercise, and my preferred way to move is to go for a nice long walk listening to a podcast. But even then, I can skip days (and maybe even weeks, oops). Reframing my exercise walk (which is what I used to call a long walk) to a beauty walk has increased the attractiveness of going for a walk for me.

On a beauty walk you will get fresh air into your lungs, vitamin D on your skin and the blood pumping through your body. What could bring more beauty into your life than this?

Beauty water

Everywhere you turn you are told it's good to drink more water. One lady I watched on YouTube drank four litres (one gallon) every. single. day. I think I drink more than most but it would still 'only' be around two litres a day and sometimes if I'm not mindful of it the grand total could be closer to a litre (one quart).

But I remember the glow of that lady on YouTube and vowed to drink more water too. And that's when I renamed water as beauty water to entice myself to drink up. Sipping beauty water, I can feel every cell plumping up with hydration, and my skin becoming more radiant.

To make sure that I am getting enough beauty water I have put little measures into place. At my writing desk I used to have a glass that I'd refill often. It seemed that every time I looked at the glass it was empty. But the worry of a cat knocking it over prevented me from having an extra-large glass of water on my desk. I then had the idea to buy a large water bottle with a lid and straw that wouldn't spill even if they did knock it over.

I love this water bottle and it goes everywhere with me at home. Being one litre (a quart) in size makes it easy for me to measure how much I've had. I also take this bottle to bed with me and will have drunk at least half of it by the morning, and as soon as I get up I drink the rest.

Whenever I go out, even for a short trip to the supermarket, I take a smaller 800ml (27 ounce) drink bottle which fits in the cup holder of my car. Whenever I don't, I always get thirsty. If I notice it's still quite full when I am driving home, I make sure to finish it before I turn into the gate.

I love the analogy of a plant that has been watered versus one that hasn't. The watered plant is lush and abundant with plumped up bright green leaves, whereas the dry plant is withered and brittle.

If you always have water to hand, you'll drink it. If you don't, you'll likely forget to. And you don't want to miss out on your beauty water!

Beauty thoughts

I have been working on positive thinking for years and mostly it comes naturally to me now, but there can always be improvements. When a concept goes a little stale for me even though I love it and have been gaining great results, it's fun to refresh things.

Thinking beautiful thoughts sounds appealing and helps me remember gratitude as I notice everything around me that I am so lucky to have and be a part of.

Having 'beauty thoughts' as a mantra also helps me to enjoy the magic in my life. Who said everything must be practical? Physically we are 'of' this world, but our minds don't have to be.

I find that when I start thinking like everyone else - reading the newspaper to keep in touch, talking about the bad news, complaining about grocery and fuel prices rising, gossiping about others... urgh, so dull, and I can feel my frequency lowering by the second.

That's why I love to disappear into my own little world and inspire myself to do great things. It's my sanity preserver.

We all have to live in the real world, yes, I agree (and there will be people around who love to remind us of that), but we don't have to be OF the real world. Here's what I mean: you can function in the real world and do whatever needs to be done, but your head doesn't need to be dragged down to that level as well.

Your mind is your most precious thing. Treat her like a queen and protect her from the harsh realities of everyday life. Fix the things you can fix and send love to the rest.

Thirty Chic Days inspirational ideas:

Think about areas in your life that are constant bothers, whether big or small. Can you rename them in a way that makes **self-discipline more effortless**?

Words can change the way you think and act. Why else would companies pay the big bucks to advertising agencies to write copy and promote products in their best possible light? Because it works.

Even if the advertising industry has changed because of the Internet, our minds haven't. We are still drawn to beauty and ease, comfort and luxury. Imagine if you chose any of these **as a reframing word**. How delicious!

Have fun brainstorming words for yourself and all the ideas they bring up. You might **choose a different word** for each area of your life; that sounds like a fantastic plan to me too.

Day 22
French Friday

Back in the 'old days' of the Internet before blogs were invented and Facebook, Twitter and Instagram did not exist, I belonged to a Yahoo group called French Chic. It was a forum where women like me went to discuss how to live a French-inspired life. We all found each other because we loved the same things. That group still exists; however, the early days were its heyday when our energies and attention were not split in many different online directions.

One of the things I remember fondly from the French Chic group were French Fridays. Members would share their ideas for incorporating something small and 'French' into their lives once a week. Of course, you could do this every day if you wanted to (and we often did!) but French Friday was a fun focus to try things such as:

- Upgrading one aspect of your grooming - painting your nails if you normally didn't, trying a new hairstyle, or practicing your eye makeup

- Taking a pretty cloth napkin and real dinnerware to eat your lunch at work

- Playing French music to put you in a stylish and elegant headspace

- Reading a chapter of a French lifestyle book and putting one new idea into practice

- Reading a novel translated from the French language

- Teaching yourself a new scarf-tying technique (YouTube has so many!)

- Going to a makeup counter to update your look

- Buying or picking some flowers for your bedroom or living area

- Caring for your clothes – shaving bobbles off a knit top, sewing buttons back on, or polishing your shoes

- Trying a new recipe

- Mastering a French dish such as an omelette or vinaigrette

- Clearing out your closet of anything that is frumpy, unflattering or uncomfortable

- Curating a capsule to wear for the next week, of clothes you imagine your ideal French persona dressing in, accessories included

- A whole day in which you eat real foods – no snacking and no processed foods. Think fruit, vegetables, cheese, butter, good quality bread, eggs, fresh fish...

Little areas that you'd like to 'fix' such as putting together more stylish outfits or eating better can be effortlessly worked on by making tiny and fun changes over time.

When I've tried to massively overhaul my life in every way all at once it usually ends in abject failure simply because there are too many balls in the air to keep a track of. It becomes exhausting and I give up, going back to my old ways which, even if I am unhappy with, are comforting and familiar.

My favourite way to upgrade areas of my life is like the concept of French Friday – small enjoyable changes that don't cost anything yet add so much value to my life.

A no-spend or low-spend Friday

The French are famously frugal, not wasting money with unnecessary or excessive spending. Maybe this will change over time with globalization, but it used to be that the French, along with other European countries, valued good quality and the correct number of possessions for their desired lifestyle.

In addition, French homes are usually quite small so there is not as much room for 'stuff' as there is in countries such as the United States, where homes are often large and relatively cheap.

In New Zealand we are more like the French; housing is expensive and often small. However, this too is changing. Homes are getting bigger and many people are lured into shopping up large and buying everything they could ever want regardless of whether they can afford it or not.

In this environment it is harder to be discerning and live with a small, curated household than it is to live in a shop-shop-shop way that leaves your house cluttered and your bank account overdrawn. We are bombarded with advertising, emails and sales every week to entice us to spend.

Now imagine a French Friday where you'd scrutinize your spending for the day. Every time you reached for your wallet, you'd ask yourself if your Parisian alter ego would buy that item. Maybe you can imagine your French self enjoying an espresso at an independent café, but not buying fast food for lunch.

Instead you've made a rocket salad at home with leftover roast chicken, avocado (mashed with lemon juice to keep it green) and a tiny pottle of extra virgin olive oil for dressing. You plan to purchase a fresh bakery bread roll on the day to pair it with.

In this scenario you have chosen to be thoughtful with your spending, your health and your pleasure.

If you've given yourself a treat budget of, say, $5 that would cover the coffee and bread roll; or if you've decided on a no-spend day you could sip your coffee at home with a magazine and bring a piece of baguette to work to have with your lunch.

I used to buy a baguette fresh, portion it up and then freeze the pieces in a Ziploc bag. Each morning I would take a serving from the freezer and my bread would be perfect by lunchtime. I have found that when you freeze bread straight away it tastes just as fresh when thawed. The French may frown on this, but some things you have to be practical about and this way worked for me.

In your lunch break, instead of strolling aimlessly around the shops to see what you can buy, you might have a specific item you've been needing so you research that to make the best choice. Or, you skip the shops altogether and walk through the park instead, enjoying the green space as a break in your artificially lit day.

In the evening you could invite friends over for a casual dinner with wine instead of going out to eat. People don't need fancy food to be happy; it's more about the ambience. Choose a main course that you cook a lot so that you know it will work out (which is a roast for us), a cheese platter to start with and a simple dessert (I often make apple crumble) or even a dessert platter with dark chocolate and other sweet goodies for guests to nibble on.

It's a great pattern interrupt to give yourself a fun challenge such as a no-spend or low-spend day. By asking yourself, 'How can I most enjoy my French Friday without touching my wallet?' you will start to come up with the most inspired ideas.

When I've cooked a pantry meal instead of rushing to the supermarket, I've made dinners that my husband has raved about the most. It's amazing what you can cobble together when you are given a finite group of ingredients to choose from; much like those cooking shows where the contestants are given a box of food to produce a meal with. But without the pressure cooker environment and the very real possibility of being voted out, thank goodness!

A pleasurable Friday

The French are also well-known hedonists and pleasure-seekers. They flirt, they wear beautiful clothes, their perfume is the best in the world and their arts and culture is at another level. Apparently, you will never see a French person rushing around doing a million things at once. They are not martyrs to their to-do lists and sometimes can even be called... lazy.

Many of us could learn to be a little lazier, no? We burn ourselves out and then eat junky snack foods for a moment of pleasure and an energy boost. When I started slowing down, taking the time to plan for good meals and enjoy reading my current book or magazine for half-an-hour with a cup of tea, life got better.

Because my meals were not poorly organized and last minute, they were satisfying enough to last me until my next meal and were far more nutritious as well. Then I had the lightning bolt thought: What if I had one day a week where I did exactly as I pleased; where I spent time doing *only* things which gave me pleasure.

And if I couldn't do it for a whole day, why not block out a half day as my French Friday where I could relax and enjoy life, doing as much or as little as I pleased? I work from home now, so perhaps I could plan my week so that I got everything done from Monday to Thursday and had a play day on Friday?

If you work full-time, you still have weekends, so perhaps Sunday morning or Saturday afternoon could be your playtime. No laundry or guilt allowed! Although, I don't mind ironing now, so perhaps I would press a few shirts while listening to an audiobook or beautiful music. But likely I would spend that time perusing my style files, meeting with a friend for coffee, or walking my dogs through the city window-shopping to see what is new in fashion for the season.

My ideal play day would involve any or all of:

- A leisurely breakfast
- A dog walk
- Style file organisation and perusing

- Lunch out
- Shopping for something I've been wanting
- Browsing around a new shopping area
- Morning or afternoon tea spent reading a book, whether at home or in a café
- Having a play around in my closet and creating a chic capsule wardrobe for fun

I'll often do one of these things in a normal day but imagine if you dedicated a whole day to pleasure and did anything you wanted to. Wouldn't that be amazing? And decadent? But do we ever do it? No! Well I don't anyway. Why? Because it feels like *too much*. Too much good stuff. Too selfish. Too lazy. The crazy thing is no-one has ever told me these things, it's just what I think myself. And plus, I'm not that organized. I imagine you'd have to have everything sorted so you could 'take the day off'.

Maybe that's the challenge then? Treating it like a mini-break where you can't tend to your normal jobs, so you have to plan for it. I like that!

Thirty Chic Days inspirational ideas:

Choose a day that you'd like to make 'French'; it doesn't have to be a Friday, but the alliteration does have a nice ring to it, plus Friday is a day that naturally lends itself to **doing something a bit different and fun**. But there's no reason why you couldn't have a French Tuesday or even a Le Weekend, where you immerse yourself in your French fantasy life from Friday night to Sunday night!

Transport yourself to Paris in your mind and do what you think you might do on vacation there. You could have brunch at a local French café, take the air with a stroll along the beach or through a park, and pick up fresh ingredients and a bottle of French wine for a simple dinner *chez vous* (at home).

If you can invite friends to join you, so much the better!

Day 23
Know how to lift your mood

When I feel good and the sun is shining in my mind, it doesn't matter if it's pouring with rain and windy outside; I feel like I can handle *anything*. I do however have periods of mild flatness where I feel blah and have zero motivation. Sometimes this can drag on for months as it did so recently.

It's at those times that I can't be bothered with all the little details of life I usually find so enjoyable, such as putting on a touch of makeup and fixing my hair, prettifying my house with productive pottering or putting together a delicious and healthy meal.

I have never had proper, doctor-diagnosed depression, however for most of my life I remember these occasional bouts of mild melancholia. I'd function fine from the outside, but on the inside I was dragging myself around, not wanting to do anything. In addition, everything in my life seemed heavy, and like I was sinking down further and further.

All this probably sounds quite dramatic, and yes, at the time it has felt like it. But I have known people with proper depression who couldn't even get out of bed to go to work and seen first-hand how debilitating it can be, so I know I have it good if this is the worst I've felt. But it still feels crappy when you're in it.

There is almost a feeling of Groundhog Day when I'm in this headspace. Every day we do the same thing, and then one day in the far future we die, and our life is over. Not an inspiring way to feel at all.

I would guess it is probably quite a common thing, and one that could be exacerbated by the sometimes-overwhelming modern lifestyle.

At these times, the only way for me to get through is to self-medicate with things that make me feel good – consuming processed snack foods, watching television and reading magazines and chick lit novels. Other popular ways to feel better are to have a drink or go shopping. Now, all these things in themselves aren't terrible, but the difference is when you do them to escape your reality rather than as a special and intentional treat.

I can remember these 'turns' (such a quaint word!) right back into my teen years, so it's something that has always been there for me. I know I always come out of them, but I thought I'd try and get back to my usual buoyant self more quickly with an action plan. I do love a good plan.

I wrote this chapter while feeling blah and flat, and as I put my action steps into practice I started feeling brighter, eating better and generally helping myself into an upward spiral. Then, one day, I realized I was feeling like my old self again. Hoorah for that.

Recognize how you feel

When I started becoming disinterested in the things that used to make me happy and could feel a sense of flatness creeping over me, I could acknowledge that yes, I've felt this feeling before. I also reminded myself that it was not a permanent situation and I would come out of it.

This time, by recognizing and naming what I felt, I came to see that I was the one in control. I didn't feel so helpless but simply knew that I had to ride this wave if I ever wanted to make it onto the shore, as opposed to being thrown around in a choppy sea. I am not a surfer or even much of a beach swimmer, but that analogy came to me and it is quite fitting for the feeling.

See what might have been a lead-in

What I call my bouts of melancholia I believe are brought on by piling lots onto myself and are a natural consequence of consuming more than I am creating (in all senses of both words, not only eating). In short, I am overwhelmed and it feels heavy. It's almost like my inner guidance system is saying 'Full up! Full up!'

I have brought things into my home that are now clogging it up such as magazines and small purchases. I have let small jobs get on top of me and the small-job-mountain now feels insurmountable. I feel behind in *everything* with no desire to ever catch up.

It truly is 'stop my life, I want to get off!' It doesn't matter that I know many others have far more to juggle than I do; when you feel down your rational mind isn't reaching you.

I would then eat something delicious and unhealthy for a temporary feelgood fix, but afterwards this only compounds the down feeling. I know that when I have a smoothie packed with fresh fruits and vegetables, raw nuts, protein powder and perhaps some superfoods, I have abundant energy for hours. And, when I eat a high-carb meal, I feel listless and sometimes even need to take a nap.

Part of it this time too, is that we had recently moved to a new house and even though we are settled, it still takes a while to feel fully at home. My husband is new in his job, and I am working out a good daily routine for myself. Change, even good change that you have planned for like we did with our move is still unsettling.

Even if there are no other factors, I believe our bodies and minds have biorhythms whose ups and downs are a part of life. It is in our best interest to work with our natural rhythms rather than resist them. What you resist persists, and by resisting the down feeling it can last much longer.

This time I acknowledged the feeling and accepted

it. It was a small mental shift but huge at the same time because it immediately felt better not to struggle against how I was feeling. I accepted it and the struggle was gone as if like magic.

Recognizing self-medication

The one thing that was guaranteed to make me feel better was eating. I would subconsciously start to self-medicate with my favoured processed carb foods which was a fun release at the time.

As we all know, eating comfort food helps you feel better temporarily, but you feel awful afterwards, maybe gain weight as I do, then eat more comfort food to feel better again. This is how we can fall into a downwards spiral and feel helpless to change it.

I knew deep down that food was not the answer – it was only a Band-Aid, so my first step was to stop buying junky foods. When I'm feeling good I don't usually keep much (or any) in the house, but at times like this I'd buy chocolate, potato chips, sweets and kettle corn and eat it every day, but the only time it feels good is when it's in my mouth. After that it's all downhill, starting with remorse and ending with nothing fitting me. This is not a good road to go down!

Give yourself a little TLC

I committed to treating myself gently as if I were a mother looking after her child, and feeding her nourishing food for breakfast, lunch and dinner. Making the decision to choose fresh, real food goes a long way towards feeling better.

Often when I'd go to put together a meal I'd unhelpfully ask myself, 'Do I feel like that healthy meal, or shall I go for the fun (and unhealthy) option?' and you know which one my inner two-year-old would choose.

If you were looking after a family member, what would you feed them? Something light, delicious, filling and healthy? Then make that meal for yourself. Cook as if you are cooking for someone you care for, then eat that meal as if someone who loves you has made it for you. Remove your emotion from the decision-making process.

I don't ask myself what I feel like for a meal at these times, I simply make it even if it seems unbearably boring at the time and I'd rather have something processed instead. I know I'll feel better after eating a 'boring' nutritious meal – no-one ever died from food-boredom but I'm sure they have from junk food. And: when it comes time to eat that boring healthy meal? It's delicious!

Consuming vs. creating

Something else I have identified when I am feeling flat is that I am consuming more than I am creating. Let me explain. Consumption for me comes in the form of television, eating, reading, listening to podcasts, audiobooks and interviews.

When I indulge too much in this at the expense of my own creativity, I can get bogged down. It feels overwhelming and heavy. Once I sight this and actively take small steps towards creation I start to feel better. It's a matter of doing the opposite to all the consumption activities above, one baby step at a time:

- *Cooking healthy food instead of eating pre-made junk*
- *Doing something productive such as weeding the garden or washing a load of laundry instead of sitting on the computer browsing*
- *Writing my own inspiration instead of passively viewing other peoples*
- *Sewing or mending clothes instead of watching television*
- *Writing on my latest book instead of searching for yet another Kindle book to buy (I have millions I haven't read yet already!)*

Instead of taking everything in passively, I make myself do something. Switch off the television, roll up the potato chip packet and grab a glass of water instead. Choose one thing in my line of sight that needs doing and do it. Find another, and another. Choose the easiest thing first and create my own momentum snowball.

I found myself physically tired at this time too and knew that I had to rest. Instead of staying up late after dinner doing nothing in particular (except perhaps feel sorry for myself because I couldn't get motivated), I'd go to bed. I'd have a deliciously early night, with extra credit for writing a page in my journal, answering questions such as:

What advice would I give to a friend who feels as I do at the moment?

What does my higher self say I need right now?

If I was holding the hand of the five-year old me, what would I tell her?

If all of this sounds familiar to you, know that how you are feeling doesn't mean you are permanently broken, only that you are a little bit tired and overwhelmed. You need a rest to get excited about your life again, because when you feel inspired by life, you can do amazing things.

I started being good to myself with early nights, enforced healthy meals and herbal tea instead of chocolate. It was hard to do at the time – I had to use tough love – but before too long I started feeling like my old happy self again.

What would the fun, happy, energetic you choose?

In one of my journaling sessions I asked myself what would be some enjoyable, beneficial activities I could gift myself. I worked out that you need to do fun things every day. Not fun things that give you remorse, but fun things that make you feel good afterwards as well. I'm talking about:

Doing some gentle exercise

Drinking lots of cool, clear water

Eating fresh, nourishing food

Loving your loved ones – family, friends and pets

Having a swim – the sea, a pool, a spa

Sex!

Sunbathing – even for five minutes with your face turned to the sun

Create something – a meal, crochet, picking flowers from the garden

Laugh hard at something silly

Sleep – extra-long at night or a nap in the afternoon

You know from experience that this blah feeling passes – it always does. It's quite normal too. You are a human being with hormones, rhythmic biological cycles – there are so many moving parts. You have self-medicated with food or something else in the past – maybe even yesterday – and that's okay. Forgive yourself. Look to the future, move forward and smother yourself with love. Creating your life is all about handling the everyday.

We are not robots. We are humans with feelings, emotions and all sorts of other complex workings. We are not set-and-forget like a washing machine.

I often overlook this and think for me that's why I have periods of downness. I whip myself like a horse in a race and one day when I've had enough I lie down in protest.

Imagine if we treated ourselves well all the time. *Listened* to ourselves, really listened. Everything we ever need to know is within, if only we'd listen! But too often we ride over those subtle messages because we don't want to let people down.

What if instead we honoured ourselves and our wishes. Of course, we have to co-exist with others. We choose to spend our lives with people, not live like a hermit in the bush (though when we are feeling in a funk, this *does* sound appealing). We must honour those people too, but we are doing ourselves no favours if we put everyone else first and forget about ourselves. We need to work out what a life of joy looks like for us and start living it.

Thirty Chic Days inspirational ideas:

If you find yourself feeling flat and blah about your life, read through this chapter again and follow the steps for yourself.

1. Recognize that you are feeling different to usual and name it – e.g. 'I am feeling flat and have done for a month now'.

2. Ask yourself what could have been a lead-in to the way you are feeling – post-vacation comedown or perhaps you've just finished a big project and you have nothing else lined up? Seasonal blues? You've been burning the candle at both ends? There doesn't always have to be a reason, but there often is for me.

3. Cut the behaviour off that is making you unhappy right now – don't bring junk food or drinks into the house or give your credit card to someone trustworthy temporarily (and delete your card details from shopping websites).

4. Exchange consumption activities for creation activities, no matter how small the swaps. List down all the ways you are consuming unhappily and take the opposite as a starting point.

5. Journal inspiration for yourself as if you were advising a friend and see what comes up.

6. Make a list of beneficial activities that the upbeat, energetic you might do. Choose one of these things to start doing daily, even if only for five minutes. Tick it off on a calendar if you need to.

7. Have forgiveness for treating yourself like you are a machine, and start being kind instead.

8. Prepare simple, nutritious meals even if they are the last thing you feel like. Make them ahead of time so you don't have any decision-making right at mealtime.

9. Heap self-care on yourself – plenty of sleep and rest, and fun activities that you enjoy such as reading and crafting. Think back to pastimes you loved in the past or even as a child, and pick one up again.

10. Look to the future and see what could make your life sparkly and enticing again. Could you plan a mini-break or a beach vacation to look forward to down the track? I find that having something to look forward to gives me a real boost.

11. Living in alignment with your inner desires is the only way to be. Journal your 'perfect day' and let your mind overflow with outrageous details. Be excited about what is to come and know that you can create the kind of life that makes you eager to get up in the morning and start each day. What is in your perfect day that you can bring into your

reality right now?

Now, you might not feel like doing *any* of these steps if you are feeling low, so you have to treat yourself like a child who is in your care and be the loving parent who knows what she needs more than she does. The first movements in a positive direction are the hardest, but once you get going it will become easier. Just take tiny steps.

Note: this chapter was written by me as someone who has never been to the doctor for depression, as I mentioned. If you feel that yours is far more serious than a mild period of feeling flat, I encourage you to seek professional medical help. There is no shame in doing this. As someone close to me who has suffered from depression said: *'It's like having a broken leg, except you can't see it. But just because it's not physical, doesn't mean it's not a real thing.'*

Day 24

How to love where you live

One of my blog readers wrote to me and said how much she envied my lifestyle living in New Zealand. She had visited my country once before and could not get over how 'stunning, peaceful, gorgeous, innocent, untouched, pristine, pure and heavenly' New Zealand was.

Even though she said she knew better, she couldn't help the envy she felt. She asked me, 'How can we, who live in less charmed and magical places of the world, recreate the New Zealand beauty and peace that you enjoy?'

I thought this was such a great question (and topic) because I can get the same feeling. I might live in a beautiful country that others dream of, but I look at places such as Paris or New York City and think how magical everything would be if I lived *there*.

Bottle the magic and bring it to you

My favourite thing to do is bring the essence of where I would love to be, to where I live right now. I do this by brainstorming a big list of everything I admire about a place and how I imagine I would live if I resided there.

I love living the laid-back lifestyle here in New Zealand and am far too lazy and content to consider moving my whole existence to another country. However, I adore Paris and am inspired to be my best by living my own version of the idealistic French way of life.

For fun daydreams, I imagine myself in a parallel universe living in a chic apartment in Paris. Of course, I work somewhere fabulous; perhaps I am a magazine editor. On long weekends and holidays, I take the high-speed train down to my family home in Provence, *naturellement*.

It's a total fantasy, but one that makes me happy to think about it. So what kinds of things can I imagine doing while I live there?

Sipping black coffee at my local café reading a book

Dressing in a ladylike yet sexy way

Wearing big sunglasses

Having the perfect capsule wardrobe

Eating simple and elegant meals that I put together with ease

Growing red geraniums in a terracotta pot

Planting fresh herbs in the garden and using them in salads

Playing Édith Piaf on my iPod

I brainstorm as many details of my fantasy life as possible, and it's exciting to see how many of those things I can bring into my everyday life here in New Zealand. There are a lot! And it's fun to add to my list over time as I think of ideas or see a detail in a movie that appeals.

Be a tourist in your own town

Another way to approach things is to look at the place where you live right now. It may seem hum-drum and same-same, but have you noticed when visitors from out of town visit? They bring a list of places they want to go to and are in awe of the attractions you might dismiss as touristy.

Near where I live is the city of Napier, which suffered a devastating earthquake in 1931. Because of this, many buildings were rebuilt in the early 1930s which has resulted in Napier being coined the Art Deco capital of the world.

Visitors flock from many countries to go on walking tours through the city. I see groups of them all the time, but have I ever bothered to look up and appreciate the beautiful architecture myself? Sometimes I do, maybe for a second, but mostly I have my head down driving to the supermarket and don't appreciate what people come specially to view.

In February, which is our summer, there are Art Deco festivals on, and when I've spoken with visitors (who are dressed in gorgeous Art Deco costumes, no less), they tell me how it was a highlight of their year to come to Napier. One lady I most recently spoke to came from the United Kingdom and it was common to hear foreign accents at the events. And I take all this for granted because I grew up here!

Now, Napier is not a place that gets a lot of international tourism, so the Art Deco style of the city is a big drawcard. I've always thought it might be fun to join a tour, but never have.

If you think about it, there will be dozens of amazing things about the place where you live – especially if you look through the eyes of a tourist or someone coveting what you have. But mostly we forget about those things and think the grass is greener elsewhere.

What about, as with my reader at the top of this chapter, you crave the spirit of New Zealand? What can I offer you? Allow me to share what I think is the essence of New Zealand, or at least my New Zealand, and you can see how many of these points you can recreate for yourself where you live.

Enjoying a laid-back lifestyle rather than always on the go-go-go

Creative and artsy

Enjoying the outdoors by going to the beach or river with a picnic

Dining outside and having an indoor-outdoor lifestyle at home

A do-it-yourself mentality – making and mending things

Eating meals from the barbeque all summer

Enjoying the simple things in life, perhaps laying outside on the grass with a book

An outdoorsy lifestyle such as cycling on cycle trails

Going wine tasting at a vineyard on a Saturday afternoon

Having friends around for a simple dinner and drinks rather than going to a restaurant

I'm not sure how unique these are to New Zealand; to me it seems like they could be from anywhere. Perhaps a better exercise is to ask what New Zealand says to you.

What details have you picked up from television programs and movies, books, news and magazine articles, and my blog if you read it. What details stand out and captivate you, making you think, 'I wish that was my reality'. Write all those down and find out how many of them you can activate for yourself.

Say you love the *Lord of the Rings* movies (which

were filmed in New Zealand, and the Hobbiton movie set is a big tourist attraction here). What I remember most about those movies is that they were forever tromping across grassy slopes. Is there somewhere close to you where you can do a hike or a bushwalk one weekend?

It's not that you are trying to copy the movie, but by doing something like this you are bringing the feeling of the movie and the place to you.

Travel there through books and magazines

I love to read books set in a place I adore – fiction where the main character lives in (or travels to) Paris, London or New York is my happy place. Immersing myself in a story is almost like I've lived in that city myself. It's a funny oxymoron that I love watching movies and reading books set in big cities, because I am a wide-open-space country girl where the fewer the people around me the better. I'm just glad I can get my city fix without having to live there!

If you have been on vacation somewhere and find that it's not easy to capture the essence of that place, perhaps note down everything you enjoyed doing there so you can recreate those memories. For example, I loved Hawaii when my husband and I visited on a belated honeymoon (it took us six years to get there!). The air and sea temperatures were warm and balmy, people seemed happy and relaxed, and it was fabulous to have the combination of American shopping and sandy beaches side-by-side.

A few magazines I bought there, I later subscribed to so that I could have them sent to me here in New Zealand. They weren't Hawaiian magazines specifically, they were American; but because I'd bought them there, they linked the memory of our eight tropical nights.

I also fell in love with Bath and Body Works, which I'd never seen before. I know their products are so totally over the top and probably way too young for me, but they make me feel happy with their bright packaging and pretty scents. Once I ran out of my holiday purchases, I placed an order from their website. Yes, we can buy lovely body products in New Zealand and I mostly buy local, but it had a touch of fun about it to order the same products I'd enjoyed in Hawaii.

Let your desires change your life

We created an even bigger change for ourselves with our Hawaiian trip, although it was a good three to four years later before anything came to fruition. Strolling along the ocean-front path with my husband was very different to our life in the city back at home. We ran a seven-day-a-week retail store between us, with no other staff for the most part. This meant we rarely had a day off together, and the only time we could go on vacation was at Christmas, when we closed the store for ten days (which is when we booked our Hawaiian trip for).

I truly do think that trip planted a seed for our future. We talked about how nice it was to spend time together with no shop to go to, and how relaxing it was to be out of the city. Of course, Waikiki is a busy place, but when you're a tourist you are not sitting in traffic on the motorway trying to get to work, you're strolling along a beautiful beach and deciding where to book for dinner.

A couple of years later we made the decision to sell our business and city home, and relocate to a smaller, sunnier, coastal area where we now live. It took a while to achieve that; our business alone took over a year to sell, but now we are here. My husband works in a job he loves, and I work from home as a writer.

As I type this, it's warm and the sun is shining in my office window and it's only 7.20 a.m. It doesn't feel like I have a job, even though I write daily. I create my own schedule, do little jobs around the house between times, and basically live like I am always on vacation.

This idea is a *tiny* bit larger than recreating activities you enjoyed on holiday, but why not dream big? My husband and I talked about how we wanted our everyday life to feel like we were on vacation, so that we didn't have to wait for that big trip every few years. We ended up buying a beautiful home in the countryside, surrounded by vineyards, orchards, sheep and cattle.

There was even a spa pool on the patio when we moved in. I don't know about you, but the first thing I do when I book into a hotel is look for the spa pool, so our 'live like you're on vacation' wish had definitely come true.

Thirty Chic Days inspirational ideas:

Bring the essence of your dream life to you now. Where is the place(s) you daydream about? Brainstorm a big, long list of everything you love about that place, what you've done there while on vacation, and how you imagine your ideal life might be like if you lived there.

Read through your list and see how happy and excited it makes you feel. That's a good feeling and you created it with just a few words from your memory and imagination; how cool is that!

Choose a few details from your list and incorporate them into your life today. Even if it's only simple things such as planting herb seedlings and playing music in your car, you will find you feel lighter and happier.

No longer will you yearn for that place. You will visit there one day if you wish, but in the meantime you can enjoy the essence of your dream life to enhance your real life. Merge those two together and see how much fun you can have.

Don't tell anyone what you are doing. It's probably more exciting to you than them, and the fantasy landscape is inside your head, not theirs. Nope, this secret garden is all yours.

Look through new eyes. Brainstorm all the ways in which the town where you live is fabulous. Try to look at the world through the eyes of a tourist; see what kinds of attractions are available for visitors and choose what appeals to you personally (for example, there is an amazing wool shop not far from where I live, which isn't on any tourist maps, but it makes me very happy that I can go there any time!).

Is there anything on this list that is free or you can do today? Pretend you are a tourist in your own town and enjoy an activity without any pre-conceived ideas. Imagine you were visiting somewhere; would you do that thing there? This is where staycations were born from!

Think beyond the everyday

Consider how you feel when you're on holiday or how you imagine your dream life would be. Are there any bigger-than-big goals that you have such as my living like I'm on vacation every day? Do you desire to move to a new house or change your life in some way?

Let your daydreams guide you towards living your most authentic, happy and beautiful life.

Day 25
Cultivate your own star quality

When you think of someone who is a superstar, do you ever wonder just how that happened? What made George Clooney the way he is? Audrey Hepburn? Martha Stewart? You will likely find there are also people you know in real life who have that indefinable quality which makes them stand out amongst others.

In this chapter I will share what I consider to be important characteristics of those with star power and you will see how easy it can be to spin a beguiling and magical web of star quality around yourself as well.

You can then enjoy being a magnetic superstar yourself, in a way that suits your personality exactly. Why not enrich your life by elevating your existence to that of the highest calibre – and, I promise you, you will have a ton of fun doing so.

'A rising tide lifts all boats' is one of my favourite

sayings, and I take it to mean that anything we do to improve ourselves or our surroundings will inevitably spill over and increase the standards of many other areas in our lives too. Isn't that great news?

Now, are you ready to be the star of your life?

You enjoy the uniqueness that is you

When you embrace what is different about you and love what you love without apology, you are increasing your star quality. Trying to blend in with others and homogenize yourself is the opposite of this.

When you think about your favourite actor, singer, performer or celebrity, you will see that they are famous for characteristics unique to them. They probably haven't followed a trend – rather, they created their own trend based on their strengths and passions.

The great thing about this is that you don't have to change anything about yourself; you simply have to allow yourself to shine. I now fully own my uniqueness – all my interests that I used to hide because they weren't cool enough; loving my bombshell body type when I used to strive (unsuccessfully) for a slim, flatter-chested fashion look; and learning how to love and accept myself unconditionally.

You look after your vehicle

You know that your physical body is literally your

vehicle to get you through this life, so you treat it like the precious jewel that it is. Would you spend a lot of money on a European sports car only to fill it with cheap, low-grade gas? We are lucky in that we were gifted our vehicle, but we will pay the price unless we honour it with appropriate portions of the high-quality fuel it deserves.

You are confident

No-one can bestow confidence on you – you have to claim it for yourself. If you believe it, you've got it – it's as simple as that. Simple yes, but often not as easy to apply. To start you off, imagine doing everything from a complete state of confidence that it would turn out well. Whether you are cooking a new recipe, deciding that you are going to write a book or starting to date because you want to meet your soulmate.

Why not join those who have developed a blend of courage, daring, self-acknowledgement of things they do well, gumption and testing the waters without second-guessing themselves. When you see confidence in others it is magnetic, and all it took was for that person to have confidence that all would be well. And not just well, but amazing.

I know what it feels like to be constantly checking in to see what could go wrong, but when I decided to flip it around to see instead all the things that could go *right*, everything changed for me. I started achieving goals such as moving from the city to our dream home in the country, writing and publishing six books and creating my own success as a work-from-home writer.

Why not try confidence on for a day and see how much it suits you?

You uphold your boundaries

As someone with star quality, you have sacred boundaries. Others know that you will not accept poor behaviour, *and* you respect your own boundaries as well. It's a two-way thing. Over time you have exercised your boundary muscle and it is now lean and strong. You still have a kind heart, but you are no pushover and others can sense that straight away.

You get paid to be you

Someone with star power has often made their gifts and desires their business. They've worked out a way to bring their creativity to the world and be compensated beautifully for it. They are living the dream: being paid to do something they love so much that they'd do it for free.

I write my books and love every minute of it. I receive messages from readers almost daily about how my words have helped them. I feel so blessed that I have made my hobby and interest into my career.

What do you do that you would *love* to replace your job with? Do you sew your own clothes, make greeting cards, write poetry or short stories? Find out how you can make your passion your career by running a few Internet searches to see how others have done just that in your chosen field.

You have mystique

You are careful with how much you give away about yourself. You are not an open book for anyone to flick though. Being this way lights you up from within – you positively glow, and you find that people are more drawn to you than ever.

You forget about your weaknesses

You never apologise for your (perceived) weaknesses. In fact, superstars don't often remember what their own weaknesses are because they are so used to spending their time and energy thinking about their good points. It's not vain, it's smart. How can you create remarkable things in the world if you're constantly looking into your shadows and worrying about them? Turn your face to the sun instead and soak in its energizing rays as you focus on all that is amazing about you.

Everyone has strengths and weaknesses. Do you think Queen Elizabeth II thinks about her flaws, or does she just get on with her job? Do you think Aerin Lauder wonders to herself if people will say she's successful only because she has family money, or does she continue to create a bigger and more beautiful vision for her lifestyle product line?

Every single one of us has thoughts and weaknesses that will hold us back if we let them, but what's the point in doing that? Instead we'll enjoy life more if we focus on our skills, strengths and passions and ignore everything else.

You have charisma

You are warmly interested in other people – you remember names and make whoever you are speaking with feel like they have an important contribution. You are an expert at listening with interest, and also in how to wrap up a conversation in an easy and beautiful way. You ask friendly questions of others more than you talk about yourself.

You keep a high vibration

The easiest way to keep your star power bright is by doing things that make you feel good – eating nutritiously, keeping hydrated, spending time with people that make you feel happy and saying no to things that drain you. When you are in a high frequency you will feel light and joyful – it's a wonderful place to be and you will find yourself invigorated and raring to build your star billing.

For me, I know I've been neglecting self-care when I start to feel leaden and heavy of spirit. To turn my energy around, back to that energetic sparkliness which has me doing great things, I ask myself, 'what's working right now and what's not?' I note down ideas which would make me feel better and then I commit to doing them.

It's not even an effort though, because the things that feel good I crave. Things like early nights and lots of water make me feel amazing, it's just that sometimes I forget about them.

Other things that feel good are little treats such as going window shopping, reading a delicious novel or watching a favourite feel-good movie; inviting friends around for dinner or visiting a relative; cocooning at home and having a 'do what I want day' where I please myself. All these things restore my energy and increase my frequency to a point where I feel unstoppable.

What are those things for you? The best exercise I know of is to make two lists: the first list is for things you enjoy doing that make you feel good afterwards, and the second list is for things you enjoy doing but that you feel almost instant remorse for afterwards.

An example from the first list might be a spa evening where you put on a face mask and paint your nails, and an example from the second list might be eating a large bar of chocolate all at once.

Brainstorm as many items for each list as you can; you will then have two clear-cut directions to choose from – the first list of your true pleasures will raise your vibration, and the second list filled with false pleasures will lower your vibration.

Indulge in the first list as much as you can and

choose from the second list sparingly if at all. Crowd out the second list by overdosing on the first.

You are always looking to be better

As someone with star power, you get to be the way you are by always looking for ways to improve yourself, at the same time as being completely happy and full of self-acceptance. It seems a weird dichotomy – how can you be accepting and forward-moving at the same time? But it is possible and there is a different energy behind it.

When you have star quality you are not looking to better yourself because you don't feel happy with how you are. You have a deep and complete love and acceptance of yourself, however you naturally want to be on the path of continuous and joyous self-development. The more you think this way, the easier momentum becomes.

You dress the part

When you are the star of your life, you have a wardrobe curated to reflect the character you are playing every day – your most fabulous self. You've weeded out the frumpy, the boring and the ill-fitting; only keeping and wearing clothes that make you feel like the superstar you are. These items are still practical and suited to your lifestyle, but because you've decluttered everything that does not align with your most ideal self, you feel more able to step towards that person.

I've found this is something that needs to be done regularly – at least twice a year when the seasons change – because the frump can begin to sneak back in if you're not careful. Plus, items start to look tired, and will need to be donated, repurposed or put in the rag bin.

Remember the star that you are and dress the part every day. Even if you're only in jeans and a tee-shirt, make sure your jeans are comfortable and good-looking (they don't have to be expensive) and your tee-shirt is a feminine cut in a flattering shade. Wear jewellery that suits your personality and take five minutes to do your hair and makeup. This is how you can radiate even on an at-home day.

You take the high road

Having a starry state of mind means you rise above pettiness, jealousy and gossip. You don't have time for such things because you are cultivating loftier thoughts such as fun projects, future goals and delicious plans.

You focus on the positive, bright side of things as much as possible. Be the Pollyanna of your life and see how much better everything gets. There are two sides to a coin, and one is always in the shadow. Choose to only look at the brightly lit side as much as possible.

Being this way is not only for the benefit of others; it is for you as well. When you habitually look at the sunny side of life, opportunities come along that will have you thinking, 'Is this really my life?' (in a good way). The inspiration and joy you bring to those around you are spectacular side benefits.

You are grateful

You wonder in awe every day at how lucky you got. You love your life and are joyfully appreciative of your good fortune. Even if you think your achievements might not seem impressive to others, *you* think they're amazing. This leads you to be able to focus on what you already have and how you can shine even brighter.

Comparison and competition aren't a part of your vocabulary when you are the star that you are, because you know there is only one you, and you *love* being you. There is truly no-one else you would rather be, because you love your life and the people in it. You are excited for future opportunities and grateful for all the breaks you've come across.

Thirty Chic Days inspirational ideas:

Instead of looking at all these points and thinking you might as well face it, you're one of the minions and will never be a star, choose the one that resonates most strongly with you and **have fun working out a way to elevate that part of your existence**. Brainstorm twenty practical ways you can add this attribute to your daily life in an enjoyable and easy way.

Who wouldn't want to **sparkle brightly** if they had the choice? Even just thinking to myself 'I have star quality' makes me sit up straighter without effort; my mouth curves into a soft smile and my eyes smile as well. I imagine a twinkling effect as if I were a Disney princess and this affects how I walk, speak and what I do. *There is no downside.*

Enjoy being the star of your life and cultivate a benevolent and queenly quality as you go about your day. Enjoy yourself, you starry lady you!

Day 26
Create your own designer décor look for less

I adore browsing interior design magazines and online images. It's fun to see how stylish people live, and while I know they are highly staged for the photos, I can still appreciate and be inspired by their ideas.

However, I don't want to spend a ton of money going out and buying items to recreate those looks. Instead I curate my own style by bringing pieces into my home which I expect to love for a long time. This builds the authentic layered look I admire.

I have always been drawn to Ralph Lauren's aesthetic, in that he prefers well-kept quality pieces to something new, cheap and temporary. I also adore how he has remade the English country-home style to his own design. He has taken *classic* and *of the land*, and added a contemporary, sexy, American twist. Gosh, he truly is a master of style, isn't he?

Thankfully, Ralph Lauren home goods are hard to come by in New Zealand, which means my wallet is saved and I get to use my creativity instead. And funnily enough, reading books written about Ralph, this is how he started out too. His first store-in-store in New York City had to be staged and styled with second-hand and vintage items to get the look he wanted because he had very little money at the time. I was cheered when I read this because this is how I have been developing my own 'Ralph Lauren on a budget' home style.

I coined this décor name when I was browsing Pinterest for inspiration and saw a gorgeous pillow for a sofa or bed. It was deep navy-blue with a beige 'RL' monogram stitched on the front and finished with beige silky rope around the edges of the cushion.

I followed the link on Pinterest and it took me to the official Ralph Lauren website, where I could purchase the pillow for US$355 if I wanted to. $355! For one cushion! And it's not like you could purchase that pricier-than-gold pillow and it would set off the whole room. No, as you know, you need a whole collection of pillows to get the luxe look on your bed or sofa.

I have a sewing machine, so I thought it would be a fun project to create my own monogrammed cushion (and, with my own initials, not Ralph's which is just an added bonus!).

But beyond that, I decided to take inspiration from Ralph and create my own bespoke luxury décor look. It would cost me much, much less, plus I would have a look that was more personal to me. Sure, it wouldn't be as simple as choosing from a store, but I always find it's more satisfying – and thrifty – to beautify your home using creativity rather than throwing cash at it.

The high-low mix

Fashion can't be the only industry to claim the high-low mix; I love to use it for my home décor as well. Where we went high was in choosing our sofas. They weren't as expensive as they could have been, but we did go for good quality after researching available options.

Personally, I prefer to buy fabric items new, so I was happy to spend money on sofas in the style that my husband and I loved (well, I fell in love with them and luckily enough he did too). But for everything else, I have been looking at online trading websites, second-hand stores and auction houses.

When we moved down country to the new area where we now live, we had put a stop on any spending for home décor. We did this for a number of reasons:

We wanted to pay off our mortgage quicker

We didn't want to accumulate too much since we knew we had a big shift coming up

We weren't inspired to decorate because we knew we wouldn't be in our old home for long

We didn't know what we would need for our new unseen home so didn't want to waste money by buying the wrong things

It was a mix of these factors that led us to moving into our current home and having at least one completely empty room simply because we didn't have enough furniture. This was a novelty for me because I was more used to decluttering and trying to make our abode look spacious.

Build your style over time

Our plan all along was to wait until we had moved to buy any furniture we needed, but we also didn't want to undo all our good work by spending lots of money all at once, and neither did we want a 'bought in one day in one shop' type of look.

Our new home had two living areas, so we had to find a second set of sofas. The best thing we did was purchase these through a local interior designer, because she gave us free advice and the idea to look at auctions for furniture such as a dining table and chairs, coffee table and a buffet or console.

I wanted good quality and high style, without the expensive price tag. Coincidentally, this is the motto that Ralph Lauren adhered to in his days as a young adult: collecting items to furnish his home that were authentic, of good quality and gave a layered look like they had been gathered together over generations.

When I went to my first auction, it was nerve-racking. I'd seen a dining table that was gorgeous – old, not too formal and in a slightly rustic timber that would suit our casual style perfectly. In the end I won the auction, and purchased it for a fraction of the cost of a new table; plus, it was far nicer than a new table with its patina from many years of use.

We paid $800 for the table, so it was still a reasonably expensive investment piece and we plan to keep it for the rest of our lives; however, when we compared it to new or reclaimed timber dining tables which started in the thousands and went up to several thousand, it was an absolute bargain.

And so started my regular jaunts to the auction showings each week. Over the coming months we bought pieces which slowly built our 'Ralph Lauren on a budget' décor style. In between times I sewed cushions from remnants of designer fabric and patched together denim from jeans I had been saving up. The latter might sound awful to you, but they do look good – I promise! – and add to the lived-in, casual, put-your-feet-up kind of vibe I like.

We also went bold in our living room, painting the walls a deep, matte blue/grey and hung off-white linen curtains. From the auctions I had also been collecting oil paintings when the price was right (my preferred style was classical landscapes in gilt frames) and these were clustered on one wall for a striking detail. I came across a few Persian rugs at excellent prices and snapped those up too.

I have so enjoyed this process of putting together our décor at second-hand prices and even though Ralph was our inspiration it's still very much our own look.

Now, you may prefer a different décor style to me, and even though you might not find, for example, mid-century items as inexpensively because they are so popular at the moment, you can still pick up bargains. Just be prepared to look around, either at auctions and thrift stores, or by bidding online.

Online shopping for pre-loved furniture seemed too bothersome to me, and I have the flexibility to pop into the auction house during the week, but if you work full-time and love the thrill of finding bargains on eBay, this avenue may suit you better.

If you look back at your décor style over time, you will see how some of your choices you'd make again today, whereas some you wouldn't. Your look will have changed subtly with your evolving taste, trends that have influenced you, and financial constraints either now or then.

There is loads you can do outside of furniture which adds to your look for little money too. I love one or two large outdoor pots with plants to suit your style – red geraniums for me, but also English-country pansies; ferns, succulents or tussock all have their own unique point of view and lift a doorway or terrace nicely.

I always think it's such a privilege of being grown up that we can be in charge of our own little corner of the world, making it as warm, welcoming and stylish as we wish to, and taking pleasure in that.

Thirty Chic Days inspirational ideas:

- Pinpoint your favourite styles and influences by reading magazines and searching online home style websites (I love hookedonhouses.net for movie set homes and celebrity home style).

- Gather inspiration in a way that suits you whether it's on Pinterest, by cutting out magazine pages or writing your own list of words which describes your aesthetic. I love using a combination of all of these ways.

- Make a list of items you love and want to keep, and those that need replacing: this becomes your wish list.

- Choose your next project to work towards and then start researching your options.

- Be patient and let the process unfold over time – it's easy to want everything to be finished yesterday, but when you think about beautiful homes you've seen in books and magazines, they've likely been curated over a long time.

- As you build your look, be prepared for your vision to change slightly; this will happen naturally so be open to it.

- Work on one room at a time and let this inform the rest of your home – this was a tip from our interior designer, so we started with our living room; now this is finished we are looking at 'What next?'

- Always keep your final vision in mind, even if it's not completely clear – work towards what makes you happy and be excited about how your home style is taking shape; if you're not excited about how it's turning out, ask yourself how it could be better. For me, I felt like we needed some more pizazz, so I added luxe touches such as velvet cushions, oversized candles, a leopard print decorative bowl and more gold, which all elevated our dark wood pieces.

- You want to fall in love with your home over and over again, that's the secret. So ask yourself often: How can I fall more in love with this room? What does it need? When I asked this question the ideas that popped into my mind made my toes tingle with excitement. Try it, it's magic!

Day 27
Choose to look and feel amazing

Because I've had a sweet tooth for as long as I can remember, I seem to attract the same five to ten kilograms (roughly ten to twenty pounds). Healthy food has always seemed so boring to me, and even though I am a million times better about it now, eating fresh fruit for breakfast every morning, salad for lunch most days and fresh vegetables every night for dinner, I am still drawn to the allure of junky snack foods. To me they say *fun times!* even though I know they are anything but.

I decided to reframe choosing healthy (which has always seemed boring, even though I love the word), to:

Choosing to look and feel amazing
Choosing to feel empowered

And taking charge of my health that way instead of plodding along doing the same old thing and being surprised when I hit a bump in the road. And by bump in the road I mean a health scare or even a closet scare when I try on the incoming season's wardrobe and find it doesn't fit me as well as it did last year.

When I worked in retail I saw women I'd met through the store over the course of a decade in some cases, who were what I consider a medium size and in general good health to start with. They started gaining more and more weight each time I saw them (which was sometimes only once or twice a year, so it was noticeable, unlike when we see ourselves in the mirror every day). These ladies weren't broke and struggling either; they were well-off, so money wasn't the issue.

Seeing this gave me a real wake-up call, especially when I regularly saw the other side of the coin, of women who were my age or older, sometimes much older, who were in better physical health than I was.

I knew I was heading down the frumpy path too. Maybe that's why I noticed these ladies, because I saw myself in them.

Swap around what you see as fun

I didn't want to spend my time being hungry and constantly battling cravings. I've tried that before and it's no fun, plus it's hard to keep up for long. What I wanted to find was the magic pill – the way to make the things I used to think of fun as unattractive, and the things I used to see as a drag as exciting. Almost like a magic trick!

For example, in my 20s and 30s it was fun for me to drink wine and stay up late. But as I got older, it became less fun. The hangovers for one, were far worse each advancing year, and I needed less wine to feel wretched the next day.

I also used to love stuffing myself silly with milk chocolate, sweets and ice-cream. I couldn't get enough and would indulge most days. You can guess where that got me, yet, when I tried to stop many times I couldn't. I'd spent so long programming myself that these foods were desirable that when I wanted to stop because they were making me overweight and unhealthy, I rebelled straight away.

For years I thought an existence without daily sweet treats would be unbearably boring and dull. Nothing tasty to brighten up my day – what a terrible life that would be. I conveniently overlooked where my sugary habit was taking me – to Frumpyville, and who knew what health issues I was creating on the inside; I chose to ignore that too.

It took a lot of reprogramming work because I'd been thinking this way since I was a child. Eventually I did it though and flipped the switch from seeing the foods which used to comfort and give me pleasure, as the biggest block between myself and my beautiful and healthy future.

Things only changed when I recognized that I could have fun in spite of these foods, and in fact realising that it *wasn't the foods* which were making my life fun. This was the turning point when I was able to quit my snacking habit quite happily.

I had a bigger vision in mind too; a vision of my life in ten-, twenty-, thirty- and forty-years' time. I wanted to be one of those elegantly dressed, svelte women in the retirement village advertisements. I wanted to enjoy travelling without being held back by poor health or mobility issues caused by weight problems. I wanted to feel sexy with my husband right to the end, not settle into a companionable, almost platonic relationship as the decades went by.

Your future self is born of today

Deep down I knew the best time to start planning for all of this was right now. I knew I couldn't carry on with my 'fun' habits and magically be healthy later. When you are younger you can get away with a lot, but once you pass forty you must make a choice – do I want to be healthy and happy or do I want to continue doing what I've always done?

I used to think that I'd have to give up the fun and start being boring and healthy. That is honestly the thought that would run through my head: *Just one more week of fun and then I'll be good, promise.* Hardly enticing though, is it? I mean, would you be excited about giving up all your treats and being boring instead?

Humans are programmed instinctively to move

towards pleasure and away from pain. Trying to move away from something we see as pleasurable (eating chocolate) and towards something we see as painful (depriving ourselves of chocolate) will be hard to sustain; we will always be pulled back to that which we perceive to give us pleasure.

There are people who seem to gravitate towards eating healthily and in moderation quite naturally. I used to envy those people. They could take or leave cake and seemed content with one mouthful, or even pass it up completely. *How do they do that?* I'd think to myself. When I'd say, 'aren't you having something for afters?' they'd respond 'oh, no thanks, I don't really like sweet foods'. I *so* wished I could be like that.

Now that I have successfully changed what I view as pleasurable (feeling good in my body, enjoying wearing anything in my closet) and what is painful (feeling bloated and uncomfortable in my clothes, a dry mouth from all that sugar), I couldn't say I never eat sweet foods, but I seem to have managed to cut out the treat foods that were my downfall, and happily eat the rest in moderation.

Cultivating a svelte mindset

What also helped me enormously was to take something I found easy to do and apply that same mindset towards my seemingly unstoppable sweet snacking habit.

A long time ago – almost twenty years – I used to

shop. I shopped every weekend and lunch break and was forever vowing to give my credit card a break. I'd continually be donating items from my closet to charity and felt good about it, but I was only doing this because I couldn't stop shopping.

One day I went cold turkey because I saw that I was frittering away all my money on *stuff*. Incredibly, when I stopped shopping, I didn't need to clean out my closet all the time, and I had more money in my bank account – I wasn't broke by payday. Revolutionary!

I've been good with money for a long time now. When I think back over my financial life, it seemed as if I'd changed in an effortless and magical way – I don't even remember having to try that hard (though I'm sure I would have at the time). One day I started writing out how I felt about money then applying those thoughts to being at my ideal weight, to create positive affirmations to brainwash myself with.

Here's what I came up with:

- Just like with my finances, I reach my ideal weight in a seemingly effortless and magical way.

- I know I will normalize to my ideal weight over time and it's not realistic to think that I can reach a certain weight in a week. Similar to paying off our mortgage, my weight will lower over time with my relaxed and happy feelings and the confidence that I will be at my perfect weight one day soon.

- I no longer deprive myself, and I always enjoy my food. I choose what would make my body happy, and I enjoy it.

- I always knew I would be successful in achieving my ideal weight and I looked forward to that day with excitement. In anticipation I planned good meals, jazzed up healthy foods and enjoyed creating fashionable looks with my own clothes that fitted me at the time as well as buying inexpensive pieces to fill in the gaps.

- I don't need to weigh and measure my food all the time or write everything down to know if I am overdoing or underdoing serving sizes. I have a general idea of how much I need to eat; instinctively I know this now because I am relaxed. There is no need for a diet plan for me. I know what is healthy and I know what a portion size is.

- I never feel like I can't have a certain item to eat. Some are out of bounds because they contain gluten (and I am celiac), but as far as anything else goes, I will eat it if I want to. The difference is, now I don't feel the desire to stuff everything in because I am not putting pressure on myself to Be Healthy, Be Skinny, No Sugar.

- I feel happy *not* eating things that I used to crave all the time. I prefer not to buy them and I prefer not to clutter my body with them. I love the feeling of lightness that comes from eating well and hardly snacking at all. I'll enjoy a meal if I am out, or a treat every now and then, but I feel a sense of happiness *not* eating treat foods for the most part.

- I love going for a stroll with my headphones on because it feels good, not because I will lose weight. It keeps my muscles active, joints loose and blood pumping around. I get oxygen into my lungs and Vitamin D on my skin.

- Just like I love tracking our budget and finance goals, I love tracking my weight because it motivates me to continue towards my goal. I visualize my accomplishment ahead of time.

- Just like with money, where I naturally hold back from buying something or consider whether the price is something I am prepared to pay (and naturally stay 'slim' with regards to our finances), I make quick mental calculations about what it means to eat or not eat something. High calorie food items aren't worth it to me, but I do splurge every once in a while. Just like I do with money.

A thought that came from this brainstorming session was that instead of thinking I was depriving myself not eating certain foods or snacking, I was actually giving myself the gift of something else – something even better. By 'depriving' myself of low-quality chocolate, I was giving myself the gift of feeling good in my body and knowing my clothes looked incredible. A waistband that does not dig in or roll over is a beautiful thing.

Reading my inspiration list every day (and sometimes more than once a day) meant that it was easy to remember what I wanted while I got used to *not* having daily sweet treats.

Perhaps money isn't as easy for you as it is for me, but I'm sure there is at least one area in your life where you are on top of things. Perhaps it's housework and home organization, this might be effortless for you. Maybe it's your job, volunteer work, or being a mother. Whatever that area is, apply it to an area which you find less easy and see what you can achieve.

Why *not* choose to look and feel amazing? I mean, if that option was offered to you with a check box beside it, wouldn't you choose it? Or would you rather tick 'look and feel frumpy' instead? That's all it comes down to, making a decision. It sounds too simplistic, I know, but it's true. Decide and get started. Your life is waiting for you.

Thirty Chic Days inspirational ideas:

Look at past health habits and pick out the ones you know will have consequences down the track (and perhaps they already do now). Don't use this as an excuse to be mean to yourself though, please. You're not the only one to forgo health and happiness for the siren song of sugar or whatever your taste is.

Fast forward ten years and see where your chosen 'favourite' habit will get you if you don't change. For me, it wasn't a pretty sight. I know with changing hormones that my sweet tooth will not lead me to that slim and spritely vision of myself that I have in my mind.

Now imagine **you've decided to bin this habit once and for all**. You were pleasantly surprised at how easy it was to do, and once you are out of this habit you realize it was only that – a habit. It wasn't something which was a true pleasure for you, but something you did because you'd trained yourself into it. Sure, you enjoyed the taste, but you now know that there are plenty of other delicious tastes around – taste that comes from real food.

When I read of a celebrity who'd lost two stone (or 13 kg/28 pounds), she said she'd been on a 'brutal' regime. Intrigued, I read on. What she'd done was cut out chocolate, alcohol and processed foods. *Well of course!* I said to myself. *Anyone could lose weight doing that*. And then the lightbulb went on... It was that easy.

We all know what we need to do, it's finding the *oomph* to get us going; the motivation that works for us.

Identify something you find easy to do; an area which you have mastered and where success is ongoing and effortless. Then mix up your successful habits and the area where you desire to change, and see the magic which comes from this alchemy. Good luck!

Day 28
Get your chic travel game on

I am not a particularly frequent flier, but I adore dreaming about the trips I will go on and remembering with pleasure the travel I have done in the past.

I picture myself sipping a drink in a chic hotel bar in New York City. I imagine my husband and I strolling the streets of Paris, stopping at a *bijou* café for a glass of red wine. I visualize the stylish traveller in me wearing glamorous sunglasses, pashmina wrap flung just so, chic tote by my side. I remember our relaxing honeymoon in Hawaii and my exciting trip to Europe.

Travel planning satisfies many different areas for me: the creation of a capsule wardrobe for the trip, making travel checklists, looking forward to where we are going, and the exciting thought that I will be changed by the experience afterwards. Not to mention creating new memories to enjoy for years to come.

The fun starts long before the day of departure with the germ of an idea. 'Shall we spend my 50th birthday in Paris?' I say to my husband. It's three years away but why not dream and plan? For me, the time leading up to a trip is almost as enjoyable as the trip itself.

I play French music daily to get myself in the mood, sip black coffee instead of my usual tea, and start wearing my scarves more... As the time draws closer, I design a chic wardrobe plan which allows me to pack as little as possible and get the most amount of mileage from each piece.

Practising your capsule wardrobe

I learned from my honeymoon in Hawaii that you don't need as many clothes as you think you will. I returned with a stack of items unworn, and added everything I'd bought as well. Basically, I'd taken my clothes on a holiday and they didn't even need to work for it!

The next time we travelled: a four-day mini-break to Sydney, Australia, I took the opportunity to try the pinnacle of travel achievement – taking only carry-on luggage. I know, the trip was brief so you could hardly call it a challenge, but it was a good chance to practice.

Can I tell you though, I was worried beforehand that I'd made a big mistake, but it was the most fun and liberating way to travel and now I'm hooked. Even if we travelled somewhere further afield and for longer and wanted to take a suitcase that needed checking in, I learned valuable lessons from my carry-on travel which will be useful in the future.

Packing was something I used to dread because I never had a clear vision of what I should take. I feared leaving something behind so I'd often overpack. How I changed dread to excitement was to treat my packing as a creative project and practice with a mock pack the week before.

In the past I would have considered this a waste of time and instead thought, 'I'll have everything clean and ready and decide what to pack on the day'. This is fine for short trips not too far from home, but when you are travelling to a different climate or time zone you need to make good choices.

I gained great pleasure from my mock pack experience by laying everything out on my bed to create a pleasing flat lay tableau worthy of Instagram. I included accessories such as shoes and sunglasses so I had an overview of how my vacation wardrobe would look.

I am always inspired by fashion magazine pages where everything, right down to cosmetics and what book you are going to read are included too. This makes for a pleasing image, so it was fun to create my own. As an added bonus I ended up with a photo of everything I planned to take so it was a visual checklist for me as well.

Less clothes, more shoes

My husband is an excellent packer (although I do think

guys have it easier) and he told me his tip which goes against the grain of most travel advice: he packs more shoes and less clothes. I always listen to him when it comes to style because he loves dressing well and has good taste. He is also far more organized and disciplined than I am.

When I asked him to expand further on this theory, he said that having more shoes changes up your outfits. Instead of taking twelve items of clothing and two pairs of shoes, for example, take eight items of clothing and four pairs of shoes. This is just an example, the exact numbers will depend on how long you are going for.

I tried it for myself on our Sydney mini-break and it worked well. I took one pair of jeans, four tops and two pairs of shoes. I was so nervous to take the exact number of tops for each day, but I needn't have worried. If I ended up getting one dirty there were options: re-wear a top twice, wash it in the hotel room or buy another top if I had to. We were in the city after all.

Which shoes though?

Having worked in a retail footwear store for twelve years, I've helped hundreds of women (and a few men) choose what to wear on their feet while on vacation. You want to look nice of course, that's only natural, but holiday walking is totally different than when you are in your daily routine at home. There is a lot more of it for a start, and you are walking in a different way; it's like going for an exercise walk when you are sight-seeing.

My personal favourites for summer are Birkenstocks ('Gizeh' style), Skechers 'Go Walks', and Havaianas flip-flops for the beach or pool. You might also find pretty and supportive summer sandals which will look good too.

For cooler weather Converse or Vans suit some people or choose a stylish pair of Nikes or New Balance for more support. Don't be afraid to ask the shop assistant what their most popular travel shoes are, and you might be shown something you never would have found for yourself.

I love packing a pair of black leather ballet flats for going out to dinner. They don't take up much room in your luggage and being flat your feet won't protest too much after walking around all day. I took a pair of high heels on one trip because I wanted to look nice in the evening. I put them on and immediately realized I would not be wearing them *at all* on this trip. My poor feet had walked so far that day and I couldn't even contemplate getting from the bed to our hotel room door let alone walking to the restaurant downstairs!

In general, you may have to compromise a little from your usual style when choosing travel footwear. Not only do they need to be more supportive and comfortable than normal shoes, but you also want them to go with as many outfits as possible.

For our Sydney mini-break I took two pairs: lightweight black Nikes for during the day and black ballet flats to feel more elegant in the evening.

Travel tips from a chic French woman

A few years ago, I went to a talk by Mireille Guiliano for her latest book at the time. It was such a thrill to hear her live and I was even able to speak directly to Mireille. At the end audience members were asked if they had any questions. Not many people spoke up and I wasn't planning to, but then had the sudden thought that this was an amazing opportunity. What to ask though?

I thought to myself, 'What is the best question to ask Mireille?' I trusted that I'd ask a good question and put my hand up. The presenter handed me a microphone and I said to Mireille that she obviously travelled a lot (she'd mentioned earlier in the talk that she was in London the previous week, and here she was in New Zealand), and I asked her how she packed. Did she have the perfect capsule wardrobe? What were her travel secrets?

She told us she never checked her luggage and instead travelled with a small carry-on size wheelie bag. She said sometimes airports are so spread out that you are walking for miles and who wants to drag a big heavy bag behind them?

I was intrigued to hear her say that she had three items of clothing which she made four outfits from. I didn't get a chance to ask her to expand on this but working it out theoretically I found that you could put four outfits together with a top, a pair of pants and a coat-dress.

Outfit one: Top and pants
Outfit two: Dress worn over pants
Outfit three: The dress by itself
Outfit four: The dress worn open like a coat over top and pants

She also said she puts tissue paper in between her clothing items. Afterwards I thought what a great 'life of luxury' tip that was. Tissue paper is not expensive, and you could reuse it over and over if you were careful.

I save tissue paper up when it is wrapped around a purchase or gift and then never remember to use it for anything. *Naturellement* I popped some into my suitcase when I got home so I can pack in a luxurious manner like Mireille next time I travel.

My favourite travel tips

You can learn a lot from reading other people's travel tips, and it is satisfying when you use them, and they make your trip easier and more enjoyable. I am certainly grateful to the blogs and online articles I have read over the years while looking for travel inspiration, so I hope you get some nuggets from my favourite travel tips.

- Don't overpack. Take half as much as you think

you'll need (really!). You can always re-wear some items or even purchase a new item if you need to. More than likely though, you will find that neither of these situations occur. In addition, packing lightly will help you choose more mindfully, rather than throwing everything in and saying you'll choose what to wear when you get there.

- Take your nicest and best clothing and accessories. You've waited a long time for this trip; you've saved up for it and you are looking forward to it. Taking only your nicest and your best means you will look good and you will feel good. You will feel like an heiress when you open your suitcase after arriving because you have packed only the items you adore. It's a luxurious feeling.

- Buy the highest quality lightweight suitcase you can afford. Newer models have four spinner wheels, so you can simply push or pull them along, no tilting required. They are also much lighter than in the past which means you won't have to worry as much about excess luggage. Being easy to manoeuvre and lighter in weight makes travelling a breeze and you will happily stride along looking like a celebrity who flies by jet all the time!

- If you are travelling as a couple and do want to check in a suitcase, consider booking one full fare and one 'seat only' fare. With this combination you will get one large suitcase, two carry-on bags plus a small personal bag like a handbag or laptop case each.

- Research your accommodation and find out what they have available. For example, if there is a hairdryer in the room, you won't need yours. I decided on a recent trip to not even take my GHD flat-irons (which I usually rely on to keep my hair looking good). The hairdryer in our room was quite small and made my hair a bit fluffy, but I could live with it for a few days and I didn't have to lump my hairdryer or GHDs across borders.

- Coordinate a capsule wardrobe – there is some compromise in a travel wardrobe but that's part of the fun. Other people will be in the same boat as you so don't feel like you will be the only one wearing Birkenstocks out for dinner like I did in Hawaii.

- Take cloth drawstring bags to put your shoes in. You don't want the soles touching and possibly dirtying your clothing. I always save the bags that sometimes come with new shoes and I also have a few pretty fabric bags which were gifts. They are easy enough to make if you sew. If you don't have any fabric bags you can use plastic shopping bags. I like to take a few extras to put dirty laundry in too.

- Rolling your clothes works well – you can see everything you have packed easier, they don't get as wrinkled and it saves space too.

- If you are in a serviced apartment, do a laundry wash and dry the night before you leave. You might not feel like bothering but it's so nice to arrive home with only a few items to put in the laundry hamper.

- Take a loungewear outfit to wear in your room when you are resting. I love changing into leggings and a long-sleeved tee-shirt when I am relaxing at home in the evenings, so I started taking my loungewear with me on trips as well. An outfit doesn't take up much room and I feel instantly relaxed when I change. It's also nice to take little travel slippers or soft socks so that you don't have to go barefoot on the hotel carpet.

- Buy a small cross-body bag if you don't already own one. A friend told me she found this style invaluable for carrying her passport, boarding pass and money at the airport and she was right. The bag I took fitted exactly what I needed it to - a credit card, passport, cash, lip gloss, tiny folded-up tourist map, phone and hand sanitizer. It was great not having to hold a bag on my shoulder yet was still right there when I needed to get anything out. I usually leave my wallet at home on an overseas trip too. Just what do I need my library and supermarket loyalty cards for?

- If you love jeans and wear them every day like I do, take a black or dark-wash pair with you instead of blue denim. Together with a silky black top and black ballet flats I felt nicely dressed up going out for dinner. They are less jeans-like and more trouser-like which helped me feel polished, pulled together and stylish.

- Take a large scarf or pashmina with you. My black pashmina is approximately the size of a bath towel when laid out but because the fabric is so fine it is not bulky around my neck. I wear it as a looped scarf or shawl draped around my shoulders. Aeroplanes can have chilly air-conditioning and I love to feel cozy by laying it over me like a blanket. It covers from my shoulders right down over my knees and tucks in both sides. When I leave I simply hang it around my neck. Easy and multi-purpose.

Embrace the geeky checklist

Checklists are your friend and I believe you can never have too many. Here are three of my favourites for travelling.

A **pre-travel checklist** will help you remember everything you need to do before you go away such as returning library books or paying bills that are due while you are gone; organizing pet minders; and small things such as setting up automated lamps so lights will go and off on in your house while you are away.

A **packing checklist** is great to start putting together as soon as you book your trip. I like to write down ideas for outfits and note down items I know I'll probably forget, such as my phone charger.

And a **travel checklist** is great to note down places and shops you don't want to miss, as well as useful information from travel websites such as opening hours, whether you need to book an activity before you go and less busy times to visit attractions.

Save all your checklists in a folder or on the computer so you can keep them as templates for future trips. Your checklists can be refined each time by adding items you found you needed and deducting things which were not useful.

Here is my pre-travel packing and outfit checklist from our Sydney trip:

To wear on the plane going there:
Light blue/grey Michael Kors sweatshirt
Camisole underneath
Black pashmina
Zara dark grey stretch jeans
Black leather belt
Black New Balance

Black David Lawrence leather jacket
Watch and gold coin necklace, rings, cubic zirconia 'diamond' studs

<u>Coach black leather tote containing</u>:
Dior cross-body bag
Passport
Visa card
Cash
Book
Notebook and pen
Spare car keys
Phone and charger
iPod and earbuds
Printed out flight confirmations
Printed out hotel confirmation
Sunglasses

<u>Samsonite carry-on bag containing</u>:
Small laptop and charger
Three long-sleeve knit tops – fine black merino, silky black with drapey neck and dark blue-grey Diesel top
Clarks black leather ballet flats
Three pairs of fine merino socks
Knickers
Another camisole top for layering/warmth
Bikini
Relaxing clothes for our apartment – leggings and a long-sleeved t-shirt

Makeup and toiletries
Hotel toothbrush and small toothpaste
Razor and small shaving lotion tube
Tiny handcream
Round hairbrush and small claw clip
Towelling headband and hair tie
Bobby pins and thin brown hair elastics
Shampoo
Cleanser
Facial moisturizer
Liquid foundation
Tiny hairspray
Hand sanitizer
Small perfume
Roll-on anti-perspirant deodorant

Available at the hotel:
Hairdryer
Conditioner
Body wash
Body lotion
Shower cap

You may think this list seems comprehensive, but I built it up over time. I started with what was available at the hotel, along with what I needed. As I thought of items I added those too.

I used to feel frozen when it came to pack for a trip because we rarely went anywhere. We had local trips to see my family once or twice a year, but overseas holidays were hardly ever on the cards for us because we had a seven-days a week business to run together. Our honeymoon was six years after our marriage!

That trip to Sydney changed everything for me. Before we went I decided to get my act together and look forward to our long weekend minibreak as a chance to practice my capsule wardrobe. Now I know I can do it and with a bit of forward planning and practice you can too.

Thirty Chic Days inspirational idea:

Have a vision in mind about how you want to be as a traveller. Me? I want to embody a glamorous celebrity travelling in luxury combined with someone who is uber organized. Now, I've never travelled anything above coach/economy class, but in my mind, I am first class all the way baby.

I have my carry-on with a new tube of handcream, a big water bottle that I fill after security, a snuggly scarf/blanket and my book/Kindle/podcasts. It doesn't matter if my knees are touching the seat in front of me, I'll simply put on my big sunglasses after the flight, fling my pashmina around my neck and stroll out as if I've just arrived on my private jet. It's more fun that way!

Day 29
Incorporate chic anchors throughout your home and your life

Surrounding yourself with a supportive environment is so important in keeping your frequency high. I love to employ 'chic anchors' to encourage, uplift and remind me of the creatively inspired lifestyle I desire. It's easy to sink down into the hum-drum of everyday life and before too long you have forgotten that one day long ago you decided to embrace your own version of a chic and beautiful life.

My whole premise is about small, inexpensive changes that will make you feel like a million dollars. Here are some of my favourite suggestions and they won't bankrupt you either, thank goodness!

An apéritif

One of my first changes was when I decided that sparkling water was chicer than a flavoured diet soft drink. At first, I felt deprived, but after a while I realized that I liked the effervescence of the drink as much as the flavour, so I was happy pouring myself a sparkling mineral water. When I tried soft drink again it tasted unpleasant.

Sparkling water to me always seems like something I would order in a Parisian café or restaurant, so it was the perfect reminder of my chic French-inspired life.

I upgraded further when I changed from water in plastic bottles to Perrier in green glass bottles. I buy the large size and they keep nicely in the fridge for a few days until I finish them off. At first, I balked at the price variance compared to cheaper brands, but when I looked objectively at it, the price was still a tiny difference relative to other things I buy without a second thought.

Please don't think I am an extravagant money-waster with dollars to burn – I am not. But I have always been a cost-conscious person and perhaps always will be. The things I saved money on could sometimes be called ridiculous.

I remember one time when telephone banking was new in the early 2000s and the fee to access it was $1 per month. My personal banker told me the price and I considered it, wondering to myself, would I use it enough to justify $1 every month? She looked at me with an incredulous expression on her face as if to say, 'Are you really pondering $1?' But it's just the way my mind works!

Once I gave myself permission to spend so 'outrageously' on Perrier to drink chilled from our fridge, I now buy a few bottles each week, so I always have it available.

In addition, I drink my Perrier from a champagne flute. After getting past 'the waste' of using a glass that is fiddlier to wash, I now reach for a champagne flute each night. Sipping my sparkling mineral water from a champagne glass provides me with a *très chic* pre-dinner drink experience because I sip instead of guzzle, and drink less overall.

Bejewelled

I enjoy looking at fancy and expensive jewellery in store windows, but for me, I am a jewellery minimalist. I much prefer to wear a few simple pieces. I also feel like it's a waste to have jewellery you do not wear, so I don't have multiples of things except for a few pairs of earrings and a few costume necklaces.

Recently I took all my old sterling silver jewellery from my teen years and sold it at a jewellery merchant. With the money I received I bought a lightweight travel suitcase which I thought would be far more useful to me than silver jewellery which I had not worn for years and would likely never wear again.

I have one good watch which was a thirtieth birthday

present to myself. I wear it every day and it stops my head being turned by the latest trendy watch. I think to myself, 'That watch is gorgeous, but it I buy it I won't be able to wear *this* watch'. I love my watch so much; it's my dream watch that I will happily wear until I am ninety (and beyond).

I also love to wear simple cultured pearl stud earrings, for example, but not a pearl necklace. As much as I have tried to love a pearl necklace on myself, it doesn't feel right; I always feel a bit fusty. Pearl earrings are perfect for me – I feel chic and minimal, and they remind me that I prefer simple and elegant in my personal style.

By having my curated, simple and perfect selection of jewellery that I mostly wear daily, I am reminding myself of my wish to have a curated life of elegance and experience over a life filled with junk and clutter.

Musique

Music is another area where I am reminded regularly of my dream of creating my own idealistic Parisian lifestyle right here where I live in a small town on the east coast of New Zealand – about as far away from Paris as you can get!

When I play French accordion music, Édith Piaf, Hôtel Costes or Buddha Bar tracks, the feeling I want to create is anchored deep into my psyche. As with my other anchors, I am creating my ideal lifestyle by invoking emotional feelings from within.

Why not make it easy to live *your* most inspired life? Surrounding yourself with positive messages in the form of sounds, images, items and everyday experiences means you are effortlessly transforming yourself into the you you've always desired to be. No effort required.

Thirty Chic Days inspirational ideas:

There is no area which cannot be a chic anchor. Brainstorm a list for yourself and start with the most fun or easiest looking one.

- Consider **changing your passwords** to bring chic reminders into your thoughts every day such as 'frenchchicgirl' instead of the 'fluffy92' pet names that many of us use.

- Grow **red-orange geraniums** in pots. Aside from Paris, my other great love is the South of France. I've read many novels, non-fiction works and glossy picture books with a Provençal theme, and red-orange geraniums are symbolic of that area for me. They make me happy every time I see them.

- Frame **vintage travel posters** or have other artwork around your home which speaks to you on a subconscious level. I have a mounted advertisement for an art exhibition in a small town in the South of France and it not only features a beautiful image, but it's written in French. It hangs in our ensuite bathroom where I see it every day.

- When you need new dish towels, choose colours and designs which feel French (or whatever your flavour is). I have a few with French bistro names on, and I always love classic blue and white or red and white stripes. You use these every day and they need replacing reasonably often, so it's a great place to get a little injection of colourful French flair.

Chic anchors such as these keep the vision of what you want your life to be like in your subconscious. You don't even have to notice them properly for them to have an effect on you. Enjoy putting all your chic anchors into place and see how your life magically transforms into a more fun and inspiring existence.

Day 30
Focus on creating your own beautiful life

I started writing this chapter from a place of dissatisfaction. I had allowed myself to compare my own life with someone else's and found it wanting. I wondered why I felt so down about myself and uninterested in my daily happenings – all of a sudden they seemed dull and unimportant.

It was then that I saw I had let comparisonitis and envy sneak in. It had been going on for months and I hadn't realized it was behind my lackadaisical feelings. I'm happy to say that as soon as I re-remembered why I should not compare myself and my life to others, I felt a *million* times better. And, how I could reframe envy as a big arrow pointing out what I wanted more of in my life.

Comparing ourselves with others is such a pointless

thing but I can still fall prey to it and maybe you can too. Pointless because each of us has different skills, talents, interests and hobbies, as well as a unique way in which we wish to live our lives. Even if we think our life is pretty much the same as a friend or family member's, it isn't.

We are entirely our own person in that we choose to eat in a certain way, spend our leisure time in a way that suits us and watch movies and read books which satisfies our inner soul. We decide what kind of work we want to do and who we share our life with.

Be the beautiful sister!

So how do we let crazy-making comparisonitis get the better of us when none of us is walking the same path? Does she sneak in the door when we're not looking and make herself a cup of tea? Gosh, it feels like that at times doesn't it?

Honestly, once I saw that it was the ugly sister 'Comparisonitis' and not something real, it felt like such a relief that I didn't have to see myself as 'less than' in comparison with another person and how they choose to live.

And it's always the high flyers for me. Yes, I am ambitious to a point, but I also value a serene, quiet, simple and home-grown life. I adore reading a beautiful issue of *Victoria* magazine or my current favourite novel; indulging in early nights; knitting; and spending time at home with my husband and our rescue pets. I am a true introvert who is happiest pottering in her own space. Perhaps you can relate?

If you find that you've been comparing your life with others, what can you do about it? The first thing is to see it for what it is. You have fallen prey to comparisonitis and she will be the thief of your joy if you let her!

You may not believe me; you may say, but Fiona, I truly haven't achieved anything when I see what others are doing. My response to you? Do you *want* to do those things they are doing? Really? When I asked that question of myself, the true answer was *No thank you.*

I think I should, but I couldn't handle the kind of pressure I imagine you'd have to endure to have a life that big. I've always known deep down that I am the kind of person who values a small, bite-sized, easy-care life. I like to fly under the radar, be anonymous in the crowd and do my own thing.

The crazy thing is though, the kind of person I was comparing myself to probably thrives on having a finger in many pies and being all over the place, zipping here and there and living by the seat of their pants. To me that does not sound fun at all, and yet I still think it's something I should aspire to.

At its extreme, people can shape their entire lives this way and then find themselves miserable – they have copied someone else's idea of success and ended up hating it. I can only be grateful that comparisonitis has not taken me too far. She's a wily creature you know!

See what it is you *really* envy

Instead I have decided I can appreciate where they are at with their life and go back to focusing on my own. I can take small snippets as inspiration to garnish my existence and still retain *my* true flavour.

When I am attracted to the high flyers and their dynamic way of life, it's the power that beguiles me. I imagine how it must feel to have so much money that you could travel wherever you wanted, buy anything with no thought of the price and live in an unlimited way. That's where the envy is for me.

Then I remember that even though I enjoy travel in the abstract sense, I am a homebody and adore being in a familiar place. For me at my time of life, I can buy anything I desire (within reason, since I don't have expensive tastes) and the way I live my life now, writing from home with no restrictions on my schedule, feels unlimited.

And perhaps that's what makes these people so alluring – it's the sexiness of their dynamism, their power, their unlimited sense of what they can achieve and the fact that they're always on the lookout for their next big project.

That I could use a dose of, and perhaps this is where they are reeling me in. For I can be quite content with how I am living and yes, even a little ~~lazy~~ relaxed. I also know that when I push myself a bit, even for short periods of time, I am so happy with that I achieve. I've done it before with my work, writing and craft projects and I know I'll do it again over and over in the future.

When I think about my current situation, it's that I want to be more driven and focused on my writing. Instead of writing for maybe one or two hours a day, could I do four? Could I write three books a year instead of one?

I tend to drift with my time if I'm not kept on task and now that I write from home, I need to be self-propelled. If I don't finish a chapter today it will still be there tomorrow. When I worked in a job I had a boss, now I don't. That is both a good and a bad thing.

The most fun way for me to be more productive is to inspire myself to those heights, and that's where I can say thank you to comparisonitis and envy for the lesson. Beyond my writing, I can look at what I envy and bring elements of that into my daily life too.

Here is a list I wrote about someone I envied. I came up with quite a long list, almost a whole page of bullet points. Then, and here's the genius part, I took that list and rephrased each bullet point to be *me* thus creating a very motivating set of affirmations. Reading this list gives me *such* a buzz, and I regularly re-read it as a source of inspiration. Isn't that fascinating? Here are a few of them:

- I set high standards for myself and enjoy upholding them – it's a part of who I am

- I dress the part and love dressing with panache

- I enjoy living a luxurious lifestyle and don't hide

my desires

- I think the best of people and give them a chance
- I trust that there will always be more money
- It doesn't worry me what others think of me – I am more concerned about what I think of me
- I am direct and like a heat seeking missile when I see something I want
- I get things done
- I walk the talk, live the dream, and have created a dream life for myself
- I am not shy in coming forward
- I say what I say and never second guess myself
- I have no regrets
- I learn from the past but I don't dwell there: I look to the future and my upcoming projects
- I am disciplined in focusing on exactly what I want, and disregarding everything else
- I am glamorous, dynamic and alluring to others and myself
- I love creating my high-flying, golden-lit,

glamorous life

The fabulous thing is, you start by describing a person whose lifestyle has elements you are attracted by, but then once you have all their personality characteristics listed you see that they can be applicable to anyone; not only that one person.

A tip: If you think you are merely copying someone else, think again, you are not. Everyone is inspired by someone else – *everyone*. If you've ever heard an interview with a favourite artist or fashion designer, they will often mention their references as well as people who have influenced them.

Just the other day I saw a snippet of an interview with actress Sandra Bullock saying that she found red carpets so nerve-wracking and only got through them by channelling Beyoncé. Sandra Bullock is a success herself, so to hear her say that made me think I'm not so nutty after all with my inspiration lists. It's always nice to have that confirmed though, don't you think?

I have had people say to me before 'I don't want to be anyone else other than myself' and of course, I am the same. But I think for some of us we like to be inspired and have fun imagining a glossier, more fulfilled version of ourselves. I know I do. If only for the anti-boredom factor. Looking ahead to the rest of my life thinking I'm going to be exactly the same until the day I die sounds so dull.

So here's to each of our beautiful lives; lives which we get to create in whichever way we want, and with whatever inspiration serves us on any particular day. I'd say that sounds pretty good.

Thirty Chic Days inspirational ideas:

Turn your thoughts around. Think about the people or situations you are envious of. Do they truly deserve your envy? Or could you turn it around so that you adore your own life and take inspiration from theirs as a better-feeling alternative.

Make a list and try it on for size. When you feel envious of someone else, make a few notes of what you find so alluring about them as I did with one of my envy targets.

It's quite a thrilling exercise to do, and highly motivating. But if you're anything like me and think that someone might find your journals one day, don't put the person's name at the top of your list, especially if you know them in real life!

Then, once you have rewritten the list to be in *your* name and present tense, have a blast being inspired to embody those ideals yourself.

Be you: the happiest, most glorious and beautiful you. Enjoy being you wholeheartedly. Sprinkle beauty, glitter and luxurious toppings on too. It's your life, live it in the way that best expresses *your* heart's desires.

Bonus Day
Find chic inspiration everywhere

I travelled to Paris in 2001, freshly divorced and ready to start doing what I wanted to do. I saw that I'd been following my first husband along meekly for too many years. Travelling to Europe with a female friend was one of my first thrilling adventures as a single woman in her early thirties.

I hadn't yet started blogging on living a French-inspired life, but I've always been enamoured with the French way of living. Not only clothing and accessories, but everything: how they eat, carry themselves, their mystique and the impeccable style of their restaurants and stores.

I was excited to visit London and Rome on the same trip but flying into Paris on Air France was the biggest delight ever. The air hostesses were perfectly styled in their chic uniforms, and we were served a filled mini baguette wrapped in paper, with fresh fruit in a petite lunchbox for our meal. There were no plastic wrapped cookies on Air France!

As we descended, patchwork fields of green and gold spread out below us. Then, as we flew closer to the airport, I saw Parisian towns, streets and homes. It was quite a magical experience and we hadn't even landed yet. Charles de Gaulle Airport was bustling with travellers and signs, all in French of course. It was fabulous to be surrounded by French people. My friend and I caught a train into the city and checked into our hotel on Boulevard Haussmann.

For the three days we were there I dressed as if I lived among the locals instead of as a tourist. I had packed high heels and simple skirts and tops in dark neutrals. Browsing around Galeries Lafayette and crossing the Pont des Arts bridge by the Louvre Museum felt like a dream come to life.

As my friend and I were walking around the stylish city, a young gentleman asked me out for dinner and when I said I was only there for one more night he said with a cheeky smile, 'One night is all I need'. It seems that everything you have heard about the French male is true!

Bring your favourite parts home with you

Souvenirs

When we eventually arrived back home, I was determined to bring as many details of my trip to my everyday life here in New Zealand. I still had that sparkling Paris feeling inside of me and a clear memory of all the beauty I had witnessed. It didn't matter that we were not there for long; I was smitten. By recreating the essence of my Parisian trip, I could ensure that it would not be forgotten with time.

To help with this I brought home a few Parisian souvenirs, but not the usual kind (well, apart from my baguette-shaped pen from a tourist store on the Avenue des Champs-Élysées). I wanted to find a few items that not only reminded me of my visit to Paris, but that would be enjoyed by me regularly.

I bought a few pieces of clothing: a soft nude leather pair of pointed-toe kitten heels with dark tortoiseshell trim, a beige cotton trench coat from Galeries Lafayette, and a dusky pink pashmina-style scarf from a street stall.

I no longer have the shoes or scarf but remember wearing both a lot and loving them at the time. I still enjoy my trench coat though. It is lightweight enough that it can be worn in most seasons and I love that it adds a Gallic touch to my outfit as well as actually being from France.

I also enjoyed browsing the French chemists and chose six bars of Marseille soaps with their traditionally medicinal scent. Solidly heavy, they may not have been the most practical to bring home in my luggage, but for months afterwards I enjoyed my Parisian showers in the morning.

Ideas and inspiration

Something else I brought back from Paris was not tangible like my chic purchases but ended up being far more powerful. In our short time there I enjoyed observing native Parisians going about their day.

Men wore smart overcoats and a knotted scarf around their neck. Elderly women who needed a walking stick for stability were clothed in beautiful garments, often with a surprising twist. One such lady had a long black skirt on, where you could see a peek of black lace stockings at her ankle. She was slender and wore a dash of makeup, and though she walked slowly she was elegant in her gait.

Examples such as this showed me that you never have to give up on your personal style, and in fact it is a good thing to care for your looks as you age, not vain. These Parisians had an air of respect around them, both for themselves and others. My chic sightings are still vivid in my memory, and a fabulous reminder that I want to become better with age, like a fine wine.

Back home in my everyday life I borrowed the quintessential French look of red lipstick (sheer for me) and lashings of mascara with a touch of bronzing powder. Whenever I see a Clarins advertisement I love the look of the model's natural and oh-so-French looking makeup, so I worked out how to adapt that bronzed glowing look to my own paler skin tone.

I dressed better, both at work and on weekends. I took more care with my clothes and enjoyed quiet time pressing my blouses, which I wore with a pencil skirt or tailored wide-leg pants. I styled my hair and applied daily makeup.

I did do all those things before, but it was a different intention now. The ten or fifteen minutes it took me to apply my makeup felt more like an artistic expression, and I made the effort to style my hair instead of taking the lazy way out (which unsurprisingly never looked as good).

I bought myself a wool beret – three actually, in black, red and camel, and wore one when the weather was cold or wet, so my hair would stay dry. I played French music at home. I went to the boutique cinema to watch French movies with subtitles.

For lunch at work I started buying baguettes instead of square-shaped bread in a plastic bag. I would have a piece with my salad or fill it with my usual sandwich options. I started sipping black coffee and liking it.

It was – and still is – so much fun to bring all those little bits of Paris that I loved back home with me. They all help me stay in my chic state of mind.

This example was an overseas trip, but I've also been inspired by restaurant visits and retail stores I have browsed around. When I feel my senses heighten, I ask myself why, even if it's only about a tiny detail. Then, I work out how I can infuse those elements easily and inexpensively into my everyday life.

Restaurants

We don't eat out a lot, but when we do I often get ideas for food pairings or interesting niceties to elevate our dining experience at home. One idea I picked up more than twenty years ago, was for vegetables. I've always loved vegetables and usually eat them before anything else on my plate. I noticed that many restaurants served a medley of steamed vegetables as a side, dressed in butter or olive oil. Sometimes they would have a fresh chunky tomato and onion sauce drizzled over, like a warmed salsa.

I started doing this at home, firstly by purchasing a steamer pot to put over one of our normal pots, and lightly cooking combinations such as broccoli, leeks and cauliflower, or carrots, beans and baby peas. I steam them for less than ten minutes and only turn the element on when everything else is nearly ready so the vegetables are brightly coloured and *al dente*.

I then tip a small amount of extra virgin olive oil into the pot and shake everything around gently, so they are evenly covered. You could do the same with butter instead, or a mix of the two. The vegetables have a lovely gloss, they taste delicious and salt and pepper adheres nicely as well.

I do this every time we have steamed vegetables and it takes only a second to add that finishing touch of olive oil. My aunt, who has entertained at a corporate level for decades, asked last time she was visiting us for dinner, 'How do you get your green beans so shiny?'

When I told her I dressed them in olive oil she said, 'Hmmm' quietly, as if she was annoyed at herself that she hadn't been doing this all along!

You might like the colour of a restaurant's napkins, the fact that they serve a warm bread roll with herb butter alongside your main, or the dessert platter of macarons and truffles instead of pudding in a bowl. These examples are personal favourites of mine too.

Retail stores

I have a handful of favourite shops that I am inspired by, both in the present day as well as the past. I would go into them to browse, shop or simply be inspired. Afterwards I would add notes into my journal to capture what I liked about those stores.

The kinds of things I was drawn to were their ambience, colour palette, perhaps the music playing and also how the staff treated me. You know how some shop assistants are so attentive and lovely but in an honest and authentic way that you want to be their friend? I like to be inspired by them as well as the stores they work in. Perhaps they are dressed in the store's clothing and you are inspired to upgrade your idea of personal style because of this.

One chic sighting for me was in a charity store and the older lady, a volunteer, who was serving me obviously had bad arthritis in her hands, but her fingernails were painted beautifully. 'Well if she can be bothered, so can I', I thought. I usually keep my nails natural, but I love the look of polished, well-tended fingernails. As I type this, I have short-ish nails in a buff-nude shade with a glossy topcoat.

Thirty Chic Days inspirational ideas:

My best tip for you is to **write everything down**. When you notice a detail that lights you up, make a note of it. Whether you prefer to do this on your phone, in a paper journal (there are tiny ones you can keep in your handbag) or on your computer (I send myself an email and then copy and paste it into my 'Chic Mentors' file on my laptop), preserve all those snippets of inspiration.

I love to read back through my notes that have been put together sometimes over years, because I can see **a cohesive theme** forming. It is easy to forget great ideas, so to have somewhere to keep them safe is quite soothing.

And, if you have a blog, **you will never run out of topics to write about**, both in the experiences you've observed, but also in pinpointing what you want your writing to be about. Now that I am an author, I have a never-ending supply of inspiration for my books as well as living my most beautiful life.

It's a wonderful merry-go-round that we can all be inspired by others as well as inspire them, because I know there will be details you take for granted that makes someone else's day when they notice them. How wonderful is that?

100 Ways to be Chic

When I finish reading an inspiring non-fiction book, often I am sad to let it go. It therefore thrills my heart to come across a bonus chapter or extra content to finish off with – much like a square of rich, dark 90% cacao chocolate with my coffee after lunch or dinner.

In addition, a bonus chapter gives me a sense of value. I can't help it, I like to get my money's worth! That's why all-you-can-eat buffets (even elegant ones) are not good for me...

So, I thought to myself, what can I include at the end of *Thirty More Chic Days* that will surprise and delight you, my chic and wonderful reader. What would give you a sense of completion and happiness as you finish this book.

I decided to include not only a bonus chapter but a bonus 'chic list' as well. I don't know about you, but I *love* a good list. I love reading them, creating them and gaining inspiration from them.

There's something about a list that pleases the brain very much. Lists are easy to make sense of, they are undemanding to read, and we can instantly pick up new ideas without having to think too hard. So, in the spirit of list love, may I present to you one-hundred of my favourite ways to live a chic and happy life.

Little details that you can sprinkle here and there; ideas that are easy and require little money to be spent. I hope you enjoy them!

1. Always keep the mystery with your other half; never let them see you doing anything (such as plucking your eyebrows) which would remove the magic.

2. Sip a hot drink from a beautiful cup and saucer. Don't think 'It's a waste' while reaching for your daily mug; it feels different.

3. Use rectangular blue or red striped dish towels instead of cloth napkins for a casual French touch at the table.

4. Learn how to make soup from fresh ingredients. Some of my favourites are pumpkin, minestrone and laksa.

5. Keep minor aches and pains of your life to yourself; simply smile instead. You won't bore others with the details and you will feel better yourself by not focusing too much on them.

6. Invite people over for dinner and decide to entertain in an exuberant and abundant way (however those words express themselves to you). Have a French theme in your head and host as if you lived in Paris; I don't mean in an obvious way such as using Eiffel Tower napkins (although you could if you wanted to!), but to think as your French self. How would *she* entertain?

7. Treat your husband as if he was still your boyfriend. This always helps me be lighter and more playful and it feels good too because it brings back the fizzy excited feeling of the early days.

8. Regularly upkeep your possessions – polish wooden tables, and check your clothes for small holes, dropped hems and loose buttons. I find that when I look after my belongings it makes me appreciate them more.

9. As you put your clothes away after laundering, cast an eye over them to see if they are still worthy of being worn. Perhaps they are no longer as pristine as they could be and need to move to loungewear if the garment is suitable, donated or binned.

10. Serve a tiny portion of exquisite bread at dinner. I borrowed this idea from restaurants we've been to and it's such a nice touch. Softened butter

mixed with fresh herbs plus a dish of flaky sea salt to sprinkle over only adds to the experience.

11. Have a no-snacking or no-processed-foods day to prove to yourself that you can eat real, fresh food easily.

12. Declutter your kitchen of all foods that you cannot imagine your ideal French self partaking in. If you have other family members who insist on keeping them, denote a special cupboard for these items so you don't have to see them. You never know, they might forget about them too.

13. Put together a few new playlists for different occasions such as getting ready in the morning, relaxing before dinner, tidying the house. Whenever I create a new playlist it gives my music a new lease of life.

14. Consider a big purge of your closet where you remove anything you cannot imagine your French self wearing. Put the removed items aside and enjoy your 'new' chic and streamlined closet. Consider if you can let go of those pieces.

15. Put together an 'instant picnic' basket or container in your car so that you can be ready for a spontaneous 'let's eat at the park' when the weather is nice.

16. Embrace your hair's natural texture by letting it air dry on a sunny day with perhaps a dab of leave-in conditioner for moisturizing.

17. Add a whimsical touch to your wardrobe. The French are all about classic pieces, but they invented fashion, remember? Add a new colour or accessory that is a little bit different than you'd normally wear.

18. Instead of the latest wonder cream, visit your local chemist and try coconut oil, rosewater and other natural skincare.

19. Throw out any knickers you would be ashamed to be taken to the hospital in. Don't even save them for that time of the month. Black or navy lace is a far better option. You'll feel more glamorous at a time when you need it most, and there's no chance of marks.

20. Pay careful attention to the details of your life such as what you eat, how you dress and the way you speak. Your daily habits create your reality.

21. Be aware of how you come across to other people. I know that I make exaggerated facial gestures as I am listening which I'm sure must look dreadful, so I try to smile and nod instead. I have found that this is appropriate even for unhappy news.

22. Learn not to leave things until the last minute. It's my lifelong lesson, le sigh, but I'm much better at it now. One example recently was to fill my car's petrol tank when it was ¼ full simply because I was driving past a gas station and had time to stop. Compare this in the past when my tank has been on empty and I am running late. It's not fun.

23. Top up your inspiration often with books, your style files, Pinterest boards and stylish movies.

24. Decide that you are the luckiest person on earth and see how it puts an instant smile on your face. Even if there are parts of your life that aren't perfect you can still feel lucky (spoiler alert: no one's life is perfect, even celebrities and glossy online stars). And the great news is everything only gets better when you think this way.

25. Practice being the ideal you now – the you who is at her ideal weight and living the life that you crave. Do the things you think she would do, even if you are far from where you want to be. This is the only way to bring that mythical and wondrous creature into your life.

26. Dress well no matter the occasion. Even if it's casual, you can still have clean, styled hair, a little bit of makeup on and clothes in a flattering cut with colour that brightens your face. They don't need to be expensive either.

27. Think sexy. I don't mean red lace sexy but rather a sexiness of the mind where you are no longer available for feeling frumpy and old. You are an exquisite creation and your sexy inner being will guide your decisions to amazing places.

28. Remember that men are visual creatures (I have to remind myself of this almost daily at times). You don't have to be a supermodel to be attractive. Where's the harm in making the most of what you were born with?

29. Create your own fashion look book where you note down all your clothing items and come up with new combinations. Taking photos with your phone can record your ideas too. Ask your inner French self for guidance when putting together 'new' outfits.

30. Shake off the cobwebs by doing something completely different than you normally would. Take a few things you do routinely and ask yourself what the opposites are, then choose one to do. An example for me is that I would never think to stop at a café by myself, but why not channel my chic French girl with a book and espresso?

31. Have boundaries in place, both for yourself and with others. You cannot be taken for granted if you value yourself and your time.

32. Contrast your clothing items by wearing battered jeans with your nicest and fanciest blouse or your best piece of jewellery with a tee-shirt. Maybe you will wear your hair in a chignon with a casual summer dress.

33. Make your French-inspired resolutions at any time of the year, not only on January 1st.

34. Choose three words that you love the sound of. You might like *refined*, *authentic* and *feminine* or *Parisienne*, *elegant* and *sensual*. Brainstorm ways you can be more of these things and note down any specific ideas that come up.

35. Create a beautiful morning routine for yourself whether you work outside the home or not. Mine is that I rise at 6 a.m. and enjoy a cup of tea in bed with a book or my journal before showering. After that I write with more hot tea, then make breakfast when I start to feel hungry. I love my morning routine!

36. Be pleasant but reserved when you meet new people. Ask questions and listen. I regret it when I talk too much so I try to remember this in social situations.

37. Drink tons of water. I always feel amazing when I do, and lousy – usually with a headache – when I don't. I aim for 2-3 litres/quarts each day.

38. Read something inspiring before you go to sleep. I prefer to read in bed than on the sofa, and I mostly choose a fun chick lit or inspiring French lifestyle book. Nothing too motivational (I get all revved up and can't sleep) or scary (even though I love to read mystery/thrillers).

39. Stretch your back often so you can feel relaxed. I like to roll my achy typing shoulders against a tennis ball either on the wall or lying on the floor.

40. When your day seems hum-drum and mediocre, know that inside you are chic, sophisticated and fabulous. Smise your eyes and smile that mysterious half-smile. Suddenly you will notice that the sky is bright blue and it's only a few hours until home-time. Life is good!

41. When you come across a good idea, implement it as quickly as you can. The Universe loves speed and you will be thrilled with the results.

42. Surround yourself with beauty at home: pick flowers or clip greenery from the garden; display glossy large-format books and change them out often; use your pretty dishes 'just because'.

43. A life that runs smoothly makes it easier to feel chic: note down all the little snags in your day and then work out how you can avoid them by doing something different. An example for me is that I have been late to appointments too often recently

and it feels horrible, so I am intending on keeping a closer eye on the time and allowing myself a buffer so that I can arrive slightly early in a relaxed and happy state.

44. Feel excited about your beautiful future, which all starts with what you are doing today. The details matter. What is one thing you can upgrade today?

45. Surround yourself with people who make you feel good. You will notice that those with a positive mindset are more fun to be around and they will inspire you to be more positive yourself. Limit contact with those who complain and gossip constantly.

46. Reframe weaknesses and things that bother you as strengths. Me, I am...

    Daydreamer → Creative
    Lazy → Efficient
    Nosy → Curious
    Unfocused → Multi-passionate
    Pollyanna → Optimist

    See what I mean? Try it for yourself. It's quite fun!

47. If you have fantasies that your life would be more chic and elegant if only you had a butler to clean up after you, *be your own*. Make to-do lists for the week and assign days to each task. Tidy up and

plan out your day before you go to bed. Get into the habit of doing small things as you notice them, instead of leaving them to pile up. Since applying all these little changes over time my home and happiness has changed for the better.

48. Cultivate a feeling of lightness for yourself. It starts in the mind and then filters down to the foods you eat, and your home environment. Even the phrase 'having a feeling of lightness' has a positive effect on me. I sit up straighter without effort and take better actions when choosing food etc.

49. Keep your little self-improvement projects to yourself. Show don't tell. If you are eating lower-carb than normal, no-one needs to know; you pass on the rice and load up on vegetables instead. It's exciting to talk about plans, I know, but I always get better results when I keep that excitable energy contained.

50. Give yourself more time to wake up in the morning. Getting up half an hour earlier and using that time to ease into your day feels so luxurious. In my experience it changes the way your day flows. You'll have time to apply body lotion all over after your shower, enjoy breakfast with an inspiring book and take a little more care with your makeup. You will feel pampered and cosseted and it's *wonderful*.

51. Trust that the future will be amazing. All you have to do is step towards that every day. Being fearful of what might happen is such a waste of energy.

52. Go for *progress* not *perfection*. As a recovering perfectionist this has changed my life. If I have a day of unhealthy eating it's not the end of the world now. I pick up the next day or even the next meal. I do my best with my writing and blogging and no longer think 'I should be doing more'. Life is to be enjoyed and I enjoy everything I do so much more now that I keep 'progress not perfection' as a mantra (even everyday chores such as laundry and balancing the bank account can benefit from this too).

53. Decide that you will never subject yourself to a diet again. Yes, make changes that will have you looking and feeling better, but plan for them to be part of an overall chic lifestyle regime for the long term. Deciding that sugar is not my friend doesn't mean I'll cut it out for a while then go back to how I ate before. It means that I will choose other options that feel better most of the time and indulge every so often in small quantities. This sounds like a reasonable way to live, wouldn't you agree?

54. When you think to yourself 'every part of my life is a mess at the moment, where do I even start?' remember that one good discipline leads to the

next. So, when you decide to focus on one aspect of your life that you'd like to clean up, you can happily forget about everything else for the time being because they will become better by proxy. It's a nice side effect of taking action.

55. Make a list of French-inspired or chic habits you wish to cultivate and work on imbuing your life with them one at a time. Add to your list whenever you come across an idea that appeals.

56. Affirm to yourself that a beautiful and chic life is worth aiming for. Whenever I think it is a shallow goal, I remind myself that it makes everything else in my life better – my relationships with others, eating well, and a restful sleep because our home is tidy and organized with soothing homemaker touches.

57. What do you wear to bed? If you sleep in the nude, carry on, but if you wear nightclothes, consider if they are suitable for the woman you wish to be. There are many inexpensive and attractive nightdresses and pyjama sets, and you don't have to be limited by the sleepwear department either. I love the cute, sexy, playful combo of loose boy-shorts and a tank top or lightweight tee-shirt.

58. When you need remotivating because everything feels stale, go back to square one. Remember what got you into this French Chic lifestyle in the

first place and spark yourself off again by revisiting your first inspirations. I love doing this with my style files, and books by Anne Barone and Debra Ollivier. It takes me back to that magical time when I found 'my people'.

59. Just for fun, on a normal day when you have to do normal errands, choose a persona to channel: off-duty superstar, Paris girl, or high-flying businesswoman. Dress and act for the day as if that person might.

60. Enjoy inspiring others with your new lease on life. When you dress a little better each day and show a can-do positive attitude, you unknowingly affect those around you.

61. Commit to taking exquisite care of everything you own. Declutter what you don't want to be bothered looking after.

62. When you become annoyed with your job, flip it around. Perhaps you are taking it for granted? As Stanley Tucci said in 'The Devil Wears Prada', '...this place, where so many people would die to work, you only deign to work'. Switch your thoughts and decide that you are going to present impeccable professionalism at work as well as dressing the part. I still do this now, because even though I am living my dream life as a work-from-home author, not every day is rosy. Some days I

am bored or grumpy and I quickly give myself a talking to.

63. Build your personal style over time, much like the Japanese *kaizen* philosophy which espouses small and incremental changes and improvements.

64. Use fashion as motivation if you want to lose a few pounds. Find a style image online or visit your own closet. If I need inspiration to forgo snack foods, I like to take outfit photos laid out complete with shoes and accessories. Because they are my own clothes (just a little bit snug though), I can easily imagine myself wearing them and feeling fabulous. This thought more than compensates for the 'deprivation' of not being able to stuff my face with salty snacks.

65. Create a vision in your mind of your ideal lifestyle. Jot down bullet points and then be inspired to start putting some of those details into place. You can build your dream life day by day, bit by bit. I have a ring binder of all the glorious visions I've written over the years and it's so fun to read back through them. Some points I've achieved, and others remind me of all the goodness that is still to come.

66. Develop your own fashion uniform for different areas of your life. For me, it's writing at home,

going out on errands, date night with my husband, meeting friends for dinner etc. I love putting together inspiration to help me avoid wearing the same old things over and over.

67. If you are feeling overwhelmed, look at where you can simplify. Can you condense your magazine subscriptions? Revisit recurring obligations? Clean out your pantry and vow to use up all the gathered food items before you shop for more?

68. Don't be tempted to compare yourself with others; it's such a wasted exercise. Instead, when you notice someone who has something you don't, thank the Universe for showing you what you want. Write it down on your ideal life wish list or save an image onto a private Pinterest board called 'my dream life'. What is available to others is also available to you. Dream and draw it to you.

69. Outsource something that causes you stress. I am happy to do my own nails and most body maintenance, plus I only visit the hairdresser once every three months, however when I booked in a weekly housecleaner I thought I'd died and gone to heaven. Be happy to spend on what *you* value and don't worry about what others might think.

70. Be the queen of your life. Have self-identified ideals you uphold and know what you are no

longer available for. My queen is committed to raising her standards in every area of her life and is no longer available for low-quality experiences. She curates her belongings and enjoys an orderly and peaceful existence.

71. Embrace your home to embrace your life. Whenever I take my home for granted and do the bare minimum of tidying and cleaning, I feel heavy. It might be at a busy time or I'm feeling a little lazy and unmotivated; it doesn't matter the reason. When I catch this and 'force' myself to do a few extra chores and tidy things away, I feel buoyed. When we support our home, our home supports us.

72. What lifestyle change could you reframe in an enticing way to make it more effortless for yourself? An example for me is dinner. Because my husband comes home quite late from work on weekdays, I cook dinner every night. Mostly I don't mind being in charge, but some days I can't think what to make, can't be bothered chopping vegetables... How I turn this around is that I feel anticipation for a relaxing evening with my favourite person in the world, and I want to make it welcoming for him as well. This gives me all the motivation I need to have dinner prepped and cooking when he walks in the door. We then enjoy a glass of wine until dinner is ready to serve up.

73. I have found that excitement is the key to achieving anything you desire. It is the fuel that will enable you to make positive and lasting changes to reach your goal no matter what that goal is. You don't need to be excited already – you can literally create your own excitement from thin air. Talking something up and speaking positively about it will make you happy to be doing it and the rest will follow.

74. After the age of forty you make a decision about whether you are going to be healthy or not. You choose to take charge of your wellbeing and change the way you do things – with pleasure – or you become frumpier and encounter health problems over time. This thought helps me think beyond the moment of 'I don't feel like going for a walk today' or 'I like the way this tastes' with no regard for how nutritious the food is. Our daily actions build up and we want to be gorgeous and healthy as we get older, am I right?

75. Develop your own elegant structure for the days and weeks of your life. Ask how your French self would plan her schedule for maximum ease and enjoyment.

76. Know that how you are today is completely negotiable. There is no limit to how good things can get if you let them. I am very happy now, but I also know that I can change and improve if I

want to. It's a highly motivating way to think and quite exciting too!

77. Brainstorm ten quick and easy ways you can be chicer in your everyday life. If you come up with twenty, even better.

78. Read your big glossy picture books for inspiration. I have maybe a dozen, and they mostly sit on my bookshelf. I now take one or two at a time and leave them on the coffee table where I can pick one up for a two-minute beauty break.

79. Go into your closet and curate a small 'Paris girl' capsule from items you already own. I'll bet you can. It's such a fun exercise and inspiring too. Add the details such as a scarf or long rope of pearls.

80. Kindle your own momentum by dreaming of how you can enhance your already amazing life by adding elements of beauty and style. I find this makes self-improvement so much more fun and easier. One such idea for me is to research chic yet casual hairstyle updos on YouTube.

81. Give up being a victim. If you have ever blamed anyone else for some part of your life, stop it right now! I'm thinking of an excuse that used to be mine when my husband and I ran our retail footwear business: 'I can't go for a walk after work because we drive home together and then when we get home I start cooking dinner.' This meant I

wasn't exercising at all. I stopped blaming him for my laziness and started walking on my lunch break, as well as after work on the nights he cooked.

82. Upgrade your idea of what's fun. If there are 'fun' things that don't feel good after you've done them then they cannot stay in the fun category. I'm looking at you, milk-chocolate-binge. On the other hand, reading-a-chic-lit-novel can stay.

83. If you have self-improvements in the back of your mind that you've tried and failed at before, dig one out and write down all the exciting ways you could achieve it and how you are going to feel afterwards (amazing, obviously!).

84. Find yourself some beautiful notebooks to start journaling details of your dream life, writing your goals down in every day and designing your chic wardrobe for the upcoming season. Carry one everywhere with you. Phones are great for taking notes or sending yourself an email reminder, but I love hand-written notebooks for inspiration and little sketches of outfit ideas I've seen.

85. Being chic isn't all about red lipstick and silk scarves. You can design your chic way of living to be perfectly suited to you. My lifestyle is quite casual, simple and quiet but I love my touches of French Chic – they make me feel joyous.

86. Ask yourself what would make your inner French girl happy. Does she need weekly flowers? Times of solitude to reflect? To play with her makeup every day?

87. Choose a place that you resonate with (Paris and the South of France for me) and use it as a guiding light in how you live your life.

88. When you are buying garments that touch the skin such as underwear and sleepwear, have a word or phrase that appeals to your inner French self. It could be 'sexy', 'sensual', 'feminine', 'femme fatale', 'bombshell' or 'demure'. Use your word(s) to have a cohesive intimate style.

89. To make desired changes in your life, change your environment. Something as simple as moving furniture, artwork and accessories around can make everything seem new, and it brings about a refreshing mental change as well.

90. Know yourself and what you need to be happy. I don't need big plans and lots of outings like others I know do. My contentment comes from homemaking and pottering around the house, reading, writing, dreaming and creating.

91. A chic life is in the details. I like to notice what others do and add them to my own personal style, such as entertaining using vintage china, speaking in a soft and pleasant voice and wearing

pretty earrings. It's all those little details that make you happy and impart a pleasant experience for your friends and family.

92. Be as healthy as you can – if you don't have your health, you have nothing. We are a soul, and the body we have is our home for this lifetime. If we treat it well, we have the best chance of enjoying the journey. I used to conveniently forget about the effects of the food I ate – I simply loved the taste. Once I researched why my body felt so wretched after certain foods (such as falling asleep after eating popcorn one day!) it made it easy to remove them from my life.

93. Tip out your underwear drawer and put back only those items which are beautiful, comfortable and fit you well. Declutter the rest.

94. Train yourself for taste. What you eat you want more of, so eat more of the good stuff and learn to crave that.

95. Have go-to mantras. My current favourite is two words: 'perfect timing'. Whenever I think something like 'I won't get this finished before I have to go out', I say, 'perfect timing' and it always works. When I'm running late and think 'Oh no, I'm late again, they will be waiting for me', I say, 'perfect timing' and relax. When I get there, the

others are arriving at the same time. It works so well!

96. It's never too late to make new friends. If you come across another woman who seems on your wavelength, be brave and suggest getting together for a coffee.

97. If you are ever stuck in a grumpy or down mood, ask yourself what you could do that would help you feel better. I did this a few days ago and received a response that I could forgive myself for the sugary foods I had eaten that day, tidy up my writing desk and have an early night. I did all these things and felt amazing again the next day.

98. Know that you are enough. You don't have to be perfect; when I decided to be 'good enough' and forgot about doing everything to perfectionist standards, I felt the self-imposed pressure lessen. I encourage you to do the same. Even on lazy days I say to myself, 'That's okay, you're fine as you are'. It feels so soothing and my inner resistance melts away.

99. Get into the habit of picking up as you go. When I slip the other way and don't tend to little jobs as I come across them, they pile up and feel so heavy. Lighter feels better.

100. Enjoy fully this strange and wonderful thing we call life. When I think about what we are each

here to do on earth it makes my head hurt because it's too big a thought to entertain. What I do know is that when I create my own fun and spread that happiness around to others, it feels good. And that's all any of us can do, isn't it? Be true to yourself and embrace the uniqueness that is you. There is no-one else on the planet that thinks the same way you do. Live in your desired way of chicness and know that by doing what you love, you are giving others permission to do the same. It's our job to spread the message that a beautiful life is worth aiming for.

A Note from the Author

It was such a pleasure to write this book and I truly hope you have enjoyed reading it. I would be thrilled to think that in some small way I have inspired you to consider your own life differently; to live beautifully and well, to embrace your eccentricities and know that what you love is entirely okay.

When you have a moment, I would be so grateful if you could write an honest review on Amazon. These reviews are vital to authors and will help other chic ladies like yourself find my books.

Whether you have read all my books, or this is your first one, I thank you for being here. If you want to write, you can contact me at: fiona@howtobechic.com. I'd love to hear what chapter you enjoyed most and ideas you have put into practice.

With all my love,

Fiona

About the Author

Fiona Ferris is passionate about, and has studied the topic of living well for more than twenty years, in particular that a simple and beautiful life can be achieved without spending a lot of money.

Fiona finds inspiration from all over the place including Paris and France, the countryside, big cities, fancy hotels, music, beautiful scents, magazines, books, all those fabulous blogs out there, people, pets, nature, other countries and cultures; really, everywhere she looks.

Fiona lives in the beautiful and sunny wine region of Hawke's Bay, New Zealand, with her husband, Paul, their rescue cats Jessica and Nina and rescue dogs Daphne and Chloe.

To learn more about Fiona, you can connect with her at:

howtobechic.com
fionaferris.com
facebook.com/fionaferrisauthor
twitter.com/fiona_ferris
instagram.com/fionaferrisnz
youtube.com/fionaferris

Book Bonuses

http://bit.ly/ThirtyChicDaysBookBonuses

Type in the link above to receive your free special bonuses.

'21 ways to be chic' is a fun list of chic living reminders, with an MP3 recording to accompany it so you can listen on the go as well.

Excerpts from all of Fiona's books in PDF format.

You will also **receive a subscription** to Fiona's blog '*How to be Chic*', for regular inspiration on living a simple, beautiful and successful life.

Made in the USA
Coppell, TX
05 December 2021